SOMATIC EXERCISES FOR BEGINNERS

EASY ROUTINES FOR STRESS AND ANXIETY RELIEF, PAIN MANAGEMENT, AND EMOTIONAL RESILIENCE — IN JUST 10 MINUTES A DAY

JACKIE BROWN

© **Copyright Jackie Brown 2024 - All rights reserved.**

The content within this book may not be reproduced, duplicated or transmitted without direct written permission from the author or the publisher.

Under no circumstances will any blame or legal responsibility be held against the publisher, or author, for any damages, reparation, or monetary loss due to the information contained within this book. Either directly or indirectly. You are responsible for your own choices, actions, and results.

Legal Notice:

This book is copyright protected. This book is only for personal use. You cannot amend, distribute, sell, use, quote or paraphrase any part of the content within this book, without the consent of the author or publisher.

Disclaimer Notice:

Please note the information contained within this document is for educational and entertainment purposes only. All effort has been expended to present accurate, up-to-date, and reliable, complete information. No warranties of any kind are declared or implied. Readers acknowledge that the author is not engaging in the rendering of legal, financial, medical or professional advice. The content within this book has been derived from various sources. Please consult a licensed professional before attempting any techniques outlined in this book.

By reading this document, the reader agrees that under no circumstances is the author responsible for any losses, direct or indirect, which are incurred as a result of the use of the information contained within this document, including, but not limited to, — errors, omissions, or inaccuracies.

CONTENTS

Introduction	7
1. FOUNDATIONS OF SOMATIC EXERCISES	11
What Are Somatic Exercises?	11
Understanding the Mind-Body Connection	14
The Science Behind Somatic Exercises	16
Key Benefits of Somatic Practices	18
Essential Equipment and Space Setup	21
Common Misconceptions Debunked	23
2. GETTING STARTED	27
How to Begin: A Step-by-Step Guide	27
Basic Principles of Body Awareness	29
Warming Up and Stretching Techniques for Beginners	31
Warm-Up Routines: Preparing Your Body	32
How to Perform a Body Scan Meditation	41
Customizing Your Exercise Plan: Tips and Tricks	43
3. STRESS AND ANXIETY RELIEF	47
Breathing Techniques for Instant Calm	47
Heart-Centered Breathing for Compassion	52
Mindfulness Practices for Daily Stress	53
Guided Imagery: Visualizing Peace and Calm	55
Grounding Exercises to Stay Present	56
Tension Release for Neck and Shoulders	58
Somatic Exercises for Anxiety Management	62
Creating a Stress-Relief Routine	65
4. PAIN MANAGEMENT	67
Understanding Chronic Pain and Somatic Exercises	67
Exercises for Lower Back Pain Relief	69
Techniques for Alleviating Neck Pain	73
Somatic Exercises for Headache Relief	76
Somatic Solutions for Shoulder Pain	80

Managing Joint Pain with Somatic Exercises	84
Developing a Personalized Pain Management Plan	87
5. ENHANCING EMOTIONAL RESILIENCE	93
The Role of Somatic Exercises in Emotional Health	93
Techniques for Managing Emotional Stress	96
Exercises to Boost Mood and Positivity	99
Building Mental Resilience Through Movement	102
Somatic Practices for Emotional Release	105
Creating an Emotional Resilience Routine	108
Weekly Routines for Emotional Resilience	110
6. INTERACTIVE AND HOLISTIC APPROACHES	115
Tracking Your Progress: Journals and Templates	115
Reflection Section: Tracking Your Progress	117
Worksheets for Self-Reflection	118
Integrating Nutrition with Somatic Practices	120
Importance of Sleep in Holistic Health	122
Using Somatic Techniques in Everyday Situations	124
7. ADVANCED SUPPORT AND RESOURCES	127
Utilizing Audio Guides for Meditation	127
Creating Your Own Audio Playlist	129
Real-Life Success Stories and Testimonials	130
Building a Supportive Community	132
Troubleshooting Common Issues	135
Continuing Your Somatic Practice: Next Steps	137
8. QUICK AND EFFECTIVE 10-MINUTE ROUTINES	141
10-Minute Morning Routine for Energy	141
10-Minute Lunchtime Stress-Buster Routine	146
10-Minute Evening Routine for Relaxation and Sleep	151
5-Minute Quick Office Break Exercises	155
10-Minute Travel-Friendly Somatic Exercises	159
10-Minute Weekend Wind-Down Routine	163
Conclusion	169
References	173

BONUS MATERIAL: FREE DOWNLOADABLE WORKBOOK

As a special thank you for reading Somatic Exercises for Beginners, I'm excited to offer you a free downloadable, printable workbook designed to support your journey into somatic exercises. This workbook includes guided exercises, progress trackers, reflection pages, and more—all tailored to help you get the most out of your practice.

To access your free workbook:

- **Click the link below or**
- **Scan the QR code**

Somatic Exercises for Beginners Workbook

This workbook is yours to download, print, and use as a companion to your somatic exercise routine. Whether you're tracking your progress, reflecting on your experiences, or deepening your understanding of somatic exercises, this resource is here to guide you.

Enjoy your journey, and I'm excited to support you every step of the way!

~Jackie Brown
Fit Journey Publishing

INTRODUCTION

Years ago, I stood in front of a classroom filled with students, feeling the weight of my stress and tension. My shoulders were tight, my breath shallow, and my mind racing through a million thoughts. At that moment, I realized that if I, a health and physical education expert, struggled to manage stress, countless others would feel the same. That realization set me on a path to discover a practice that could help not just me but anyone seeking relief from the burdens of daily life. This journey led me to somatic exercises, and they have transformed my life in ways I couldn't have imagined.

Somatic exercises are a unique form of movement that focuses on the mind-body connection. Unlike traditional exercise routines that emphasize strength or endurance, somatic exercises aim to improve awareness and control of your body. They originated from the work of pioneers like Thomas Hanna, who believed that many physical ailments could be alleviated through mindful movement. These exercises teach you to listen to your body, understand its signals, and release tension you may not even realize you're holding.

The purpose of this book is simple: to provide you with a beginner-friendly guide to somatic exercises that can be easily incorporated into your daily routine. Whether you are dealing with stress, managing pain, or looking to build emotional resilience, this book offers practical, accessible routines that you can do in just 10 minutes a day.

The benefits of somatic exercises are profound. Integrating these practices into your life can ease stress and anxiety, relieve chronic pain, and improve your overall mind-body connection. These exercises also enhance emotional well-being, helping you build resilience and find balance amid life's challenges. Most importantly, the results are lasting, providing you with tools you can use for a lifetime.

This book is designed specifically for beginners, making it suitable for people of all ages and fitness levels. Whether you are new to exercise or looking for a gentle yet effective way to improve your health, the routines in this book are tailored to meet your needs. The exercises are quick and convenient, allowing you to fit them into even the busiest schedules.

As you turn the pages, you will find that the book is structured to guide you step-by-step through each exercise. The chapters are organized to cover specific techniques for stress relief, pain management, and building emotional resilience. You will also find holistic health advice to support your overall well-being.

This book is grounded in scientific research, drawing from the latest studies on somatic exercises. Throughout the chapters, you will find relatable examples and case studies that illustrate the effectiveness of these practices. These stories will help you see the real-world impact of somatic exercises and inspire you to make them a part of your daily routine.

Allow me to introduce myself. My name is Jackie Brown, and I have dedicated over 20 years to teaching health and physical education. I hold a Bachelor of Science degree in Health and Physical Education and a Master's degree in the Art of Teaching. My career has guided thousands of students toward healthier, more active lives. My deep understanding of the body's needs and my passion for education uniquely position me to share the transformative power of somatic exercises with you.

My motivation for writing this book stems from my desire to help you create a consistent and effective routine that fits your busy life. I understand that time is a precious commodity, and I want to ensure you can experience somatic exercises' profound benefits without feeling overwhelmed. This book is more than just a guide; it is a promise to be there with you every step of the way, helping you navigate your journey to better health.

I invite you to join me on this transformative journey. Commit to the practice, and trust that this book will provide you with all the guidance and support you need to succeed. Together, we will explore the power of somatic exercises and discover the path to a healthier, happier, and more balanced life.

The journey starts now!

1

FOUNDATIONS OF SOMATIC EXERCISES

One evening, after a particularly stressful day, I found myself lying on the living room floor, staring at the ceiling, feeling every inch of tension in my body. My mind was a whirlpool of worries, and my body felt like a tightly wound spring. Desperate for relief, I remembered a simple somatic exercise I had read about—a basic body scan. I decided to give it a try. Something remarkable happened as I slowly moved my awareness from my toes to my head. The tightness in my muscles began to melt away, and for the first time in hours, my mind felt calm. This body scan was my first real experience with the transformative power of somatic exercises, and it opened up a whole new world of possibilities for stress relief and self-care.

WHAT ARE SOMATIC EXERCISES?

Somatic exercises are a unique form of physical activity that emphasizes internal body awareness. Unlike traditional exercises focusing on building muscle strength or cardiovascular endurance, somatic exercises improve your mind-body connection. This practice involves slow, deliberate movements combined with mindful attention, allowing you to sense and release tension in your muscles. The term "somatic" comes from the Greek word "soma," which means "body." In this context, it refers to the body as perceived from within, emphasizing a holistic approach to physical and mental well-being.

Traditional exercises like running or weightlifting often prioritize external goals, such as improving speed or strength. In contrast, somatic exercises prioritize internal sensations and awareness. For example, while a runner focuses on their pace and distance, someone practicing somatic exercises would focus on the sensation of their feet touching the ground, the alignment of their spine, and the rhythm of their breath. This shift in focus helps you become more attuned to your body's signals, making it easier to identify and release areas of tension.

The history of somatic exercises can be traced back to the early 20th century, with significant contributions from pioneers like Thomas Hanna. Hanna, a professor of philosophy and revolutionary thinker, developed Clinical Somatic Education. He believed that many physical ailments, especially those related to aging, were not inevitable but could be mitigated through mindful movement. Hanna's work was groundbreaking; he introduced the concept of "sensory-motor amnesia," where habitual muscle tightness leads to chronic pain and limited mobility. His methods aimed to retrain the brain to regain voluntary control over these muscles, thereby reducing pain and improving movement.

Over the decades, somatic exercises have evolved, incorporating insights from various fields such as psychology, physical therapy, and mindfulness practices. Today, they are recognized for their effectiveness in treating chronic pain, reducing stress, and improving overall quality of life. The core principles of somatic exercises revolve around sensory awareness, movement re-education, and neuromuscular control. Sensory awareness involves paying close attention to the sensations within your body, such as the feeling of tension or relaxation in different muscles. Movement re-education focuses on relearning how to move efficiently and comfortably, often by correcting habitual patterns that cause strain. Neuromuscular control is about improving the communication between your brain and muscles, allowing you to move with greater ease and coordination.

Consider a simple example of a somatic exercise: the pelvic tilt. This movement involves lying on your back with your knees bent and feet flat on the floor. Slowly tilt your pelvis upward, flattening your lower back against the floor, then release and return to the starting position. As you perform this movement, focus on the sensations in your lower back and abdomen. Notice any areas of tension and consciously release them. This exercise helps you become more aware of your pelvic alignment and can alleviate lower back pain. You can apply somatic awareness in everyday situations too. For instance, while sitting at your desk, take a moment to notice your posture. Are your shoulders tense? Is your back slouched? By becoming aware of these sensations, you can make small adjustments to relieve tension and improve your comfort.

These exercises are not just about physical movements but about cultivating a deeper connection with your body. As you practice, you'll find that this awareness extends beyond your exercise sessions, helping you navigate daily stresses with greater ease and resilience.

UNDERSTANDING THE MIND-BODY CONNECTION

When I first heard about the mind-body connection, it seemed abstract and almost mystical. However, as I delved deeper into somatic practices, I realized how tangible and transformative this concept could be. The mind-body connection is the intricate relationship between our mental and physical states. It's the idea that our thoughts, emotions, and physical sensations are deeply intertwined, influencing each other profoundly. This connection is at the heart of somatic exercises, guiding us to listen to our bodies and respond with mindful movement. Understanding this relationship is not just enlightening; it's empowering.

Our physical health is closely linked to our mental state. When you're stressed, your muscles tense up. When you're anxious, your breathing becomes shallow and rapid. These physical manifestations of emotional states are clear examples of the mind-body connection at work. Conversely, we can influence our mental state by engaging in mindful movement. A simple exercise like deep, diaphragmatic breathing can calm the mind and reduce feelings of anxiety. This reciprocal relationship is the essence of somatic exercises. Enhancing body awareness can improve our mental clarity and emotional balance, creating a harmonious state of well-being.

Improving body awareness brings a host of benefits. First and foremost, it increases self-awareness. We become more attuned to our needs and limitations by tuning into the body's signals. This heightened awareness helps us make better choices for our health and well-being. For instance, recognizing the early signs of tension can prompt us to take a break and relax, preventing chronic stress from taking hold. Improved mental clarity is another significant benefit. When our minds are cluttered with stress and anxiety, it's hard to think clearly. Somatic exercises help clear this mental fog, allowing us to focus better and make decisions with a calm mind.

Additionally, reducing physical tension through mindful movement can alleviate chronic pain, making us feel more comfortable in our bodies.

The benefits of the mind-body connection aren't just anecdotal but supported by scientific research. Studies have shown that enhancing body awareness through somatic practices can significantly improve physical and mental health. For example, research on neuroplasticity—the brain's ability to reorganize itself by forming new neural connections—has found that mindful movement can enhance brain function. One study reviewed the effects of different physical exercise protocols on neuroplasticity and brain function. This study concluded that exercises, including somatic practices, promote the production of neurotrophic factors that improve cognitive functions like learning and memory. Expert testimonials further validate these findings, with practitioners noting substantial improvements in their clients' well-being after incorporating somatic exercises into their routines.

So, how can you start applying these mind-body principles in your daily life? As previously mentioned, one simple exercise to enhance body awareness is the body scan. Find a quiet place to sit or lie down comfortably. Close your eyes and take a few deep breaths. Begin by focusing on your feet, noticing any sensations—tingling, warmth, or tension. Slowly move your attention up through your body, pausing at each area to observe without judgment. This practice helps you become more attuned to your body's signals, promoting relaxation and reducing tension.

Integrating mind-body practices into your routine doesn't have to be complicated. Start with small, manageable steps. Set aside a few minutes each day for mindful movement. This could be a short stretching session in the morning or a brief body scan during a lunch break. Consistency is key. As you become more comfortable with these practices, you can gradually increase the time you spend on them. Another tip is to incorporate mindfulness into everyday activities. While washing dishes, focus on the sensation of the water on your hands. When walking, pay attention to the feeling of your feet touching the ground. These small moments of mindfulness can significantly impact your overall well-being.

THE SCIENCE BEHIND SOMATIC EXERCISES

Understanding the neuromuscular system is fundamental to appreciating the depth and effectiveness of somatic exercises. At its core, the neuromuscular system involves the intricate communication between your brain and muscles. This system relies on neuromuscular control, the brain's ability to send precise signals to your muscles, directing movement and maintaining balance. When you engage in somatic exercises, you are consciously enhancing this communication. For instance, when you focus on releasing tension in your shoulders while performing a gentle stretch, your brain is actively reprogramming how it interacts with those muscles, promoting relaxation and efficient movement.

The brain plays a crucial role in controlling movement, not just by sending signals but also by receiving feedback from the body. This feedback loop allows the brain to adjust its commands based on the body's current state. This system can become disrupted when you're stressed or anxious, leading to muscle tension and discomfort. Somatic exercises help restore this balance by encouraging mindful movement, which, in turn, helps the brain regain control over tense muscles. By focusing on the sensations within your body, you can effectively communicate with your brain, guiding it to release unnecessary tension and improve overall movement quality.

One of the most fascinating aspects of somatic exercises is their impact on neuroplasticity, the brain's ability to reorganize itself by forming new neural connections. Neuroplasticity is a powerful concept that underscores the brain's adaptability. Through repeated practice, you can actually change the structure and function of your brain. When you engage in somatic exercises, you train your brain to develop new, healthier movement patterns. This process involves the creation of new neural pathways that facilitate better control and awareness of your muscles, leading to long-term benefits such as improved coordination, reduced pain, and enhanced emotional resilience.

Research has provided substantial evidence supporting the effectiveness of somatic exercises. For instance, studies on pain management have shown that somatic practices can significantly reduce chronic pain by addressing the underlying neuromuscular imbalances. One key study reviewed various physical exercise protocols and found that those incorporating mindful movement, like somatic exercises, were particularly effective in promoting neuroplasticity and improving brain function. This is crucial for pain management because it highlights how somatic exercises can help retrain the brain to perceive and respond to pain differently, ultimately reducing its intensity and frequency.

Stress reduction is another area where somatic exercises have proven highly effective. Research has demonstrated that these practices can lower stress levels by calming the nervous system and promoting relaxation. By engaging in mindful movement and deep breathing, you can activate the parasympathetic nervous system, which counteracts the stress response and induces a state of calm. This physiological shift reduces stress in the moment and builds resilience over time, helping you handle future stressors more effectively.

Emotional resilience, the ability to bounce back from adversity, is another benefit supported by research. Studies have shown that somatic exercises can enhance emotional resilience by fostering a stronger mind-body connection. This connection allows you to process emotions more effectively, reducing their impact on your physical and mental health. For example, practicing somatic movements that focus on releasing tension can help you manage emotional stress by providing a physical outlet for emotional energy, improving emotional stability and well-being.

To leverage these scientific principles in everyday practice, start by incorporating techniques that enhance neuroplasticity. Consistency is key; regular practice helps reinforce new neural pathways. Focus on slow, deliberate movements and pay close attention to the sensations in your body. This mindfulness helps your brain accurately assess and adjust muscle tension. Additionally, use feedback from your body to modify exercises as needed. If a movement feels particularly tense, slow down and explore the sensation until you find a more comfortable range of motion. This approach makes the exercises more effective and ensures they are tailored to your unique needs.

KEY BENEFITS OF SOMATIC PRACTICES

When I first began integrating somatic exercises into my routine, I noticed a remarkable improvement in my flexibility. I had always considered myself relatively fit, but I often struggled with stiffness, especially after long days of teaching. Somatic exercises, with their gentle, mindful movements, helped me release that tension. My muscles felt more pliable, and I could move with a newfound ease. Improved flexibility is one of the significant physical benefits of somatic practices. Unlike traditional stretching routines, which can sometimes feel harsh or forceful, somatic exercises encourage a gradual, natural increase in range of motion. This approach not only enhances flexibility but also reduces the risk of injury.

Enhanced posture is another notable advantage. Many of us spend our days hunched over computers or slouched on couches, leading to poor posture and the myriad of issues that come with it. Somatic exercises promote awareness of how we hold our bodies. By focusing on alignment and balance, these exercises help correct postural imbalances. I've known individuals who struggled with chronic back pain due to poor posture to find relief through somatic practices. When you become more attuned to your body's alignment, you naturally begin to carry yourself better, reducing strain on your muscles and joints.

Pain relief is one of the most compelling reasons to practice somatic exercises. Chronic pain can be debilitating, affecting every aspect of life. One particular case that stands out is of a woman in her 50s who suffered from persistent lower back pain. Traditional treatments offered her little respite. However, after a few weeks of practicing somatic exercises focusing on pelvic alignment and lower back tension, she reported a dramatic reduction in pain. This change wasn't just physical; it transformed her outlook on life.

The mental health benefits of somatic exercises are equally profound. Stress reduction is one of the most immediate effects. In our fast-paced world, stress is almost a given. Somatic exercises emphasize mindful movement and breathwork, providing a powerful tool for managing stress. Focusing on the present moment and tuning into your body's sensations creates a space of calm and relaxation. This practice helps lower cortisol levels, the hormone associated with stress, promoting a sense of peace and well-being.

Anxiety management is another critical benefit. Many people, myself included, have found that somatic exercises help alleviate anxiety. The gentle, rhythmic movements and deep breathing techniques calm the nervous system, making it easier to handle anxiety-provoking situations. A friend of mine, who had struggled with anxiety for years, started incorporating somatic exercises into her morning routine. She found that these practices helped ground her, making her feel more centered and less reactive throughout the day.

Increased emotional resilience is a longer-term benefit of regular somatic practice. Life is full of ups and downs, and emotional resilience is the ability to bounce back from these challenges. Somatic exercises help build this resilience by fostering a strong mind-body connection. When you're more in tune with your body, you're better equipped to notice and respond to emotional cues. This awareness allows you to process emotions more effectively, reducing their impact on your overall well-being.

Data and testimonials support the benefits of somatic exercises. Studies have shown that individuals who practice somatic exercises report significant improvements in flexibility and reductions in stress levels. For example, one study found that participants experienced a 30% increase in flexibility after six weeks of somatic practice. Another study reported a 40% reduction in perceived stress levels among regular practitioners. These numbers aren't just statistics; they represent real, meaningful changes in people's lives.

One testimonial that particularly moved me was from a man who had been dealing with chronic shoulder pain for years. After incorporating somatic exercises into his daily routine, he found relief. He described the experience as life-changing, not just because his pain diminished but because he felt more connected to his body and more in control of his health.

These stories and statistics highlight the transformative potential of somatic exercises. They offer a new, gentle, mindful, and profoundly effective way to approach physical and mental well-being.

ESSENTIAL EQUIPMENT AND SPACE SETUP

When I started practicing somatic exercises, I assumed I needed a lot of fancy equipment. To my surprise, the essentials were incredibly simple. The first thing you'll need is a mat or a soft surface. This could be a yoga mat, a thick towel, or even a soft carpet. The goal is to have a comfortable space to lie down, sit, and move without causing strain or discomfort. A mat provides a cushion, making it easier to focus on your movements and sensations without being distracted by a hard floor. It also creates a designated space for your practice, which psychologically prepares you for the session ahead.

Comfortable clothing is another must-have. Tight or restrictive clothing can hinder your movements and distract you from fully engaging with the exercises. Opt for loose, breathable fabrics that allow you to move freely. Think of what you might wear for a yoga class or a casual workout—soft, stretchy pants and a comfortable top. The idea is to eliminate physical barriers preventing you from fully immersing yourself in the practice. Remember, the focus is on internal awareness; the last thing you need is to be preoccupied with adjusting your clothes.

While not mandatory, props like yoga blocks or straps can be incredibly helpful, especially if you're new to somatic exercises. These props offer support and stability, allowing you to ease into poses and movements that might initially feel challenging. For instance, a yoga block can help you maintain proper alignment in a stretch, while a strap can assist in reaching a limb without straining. These tools are not crutches but rather aids to help you deepen your practice and make it more accessible. Over time, as you become more comfortable and flexible, you might find that you need them less, but they can be invaluable in the beginning.

Creating an ideal space for your practice is equally important. Aim for a quiet, distraction-free area where you can truly focus on yourself. This could be a corner of your living room, a spot in your bedroom, or even a small section of your home office. The key is to have a space where you won't be interrupted. Adequate space to move freely is crucial; you want to avoid bumping into furniture or feeling confined. Ensure the area is well-lit and well-ventilated. Natural light is ideal, but soft, ambient lighting can also create a calming atmosphere. Good airflow helps you breathe easier, making your practice more comfortable.

Consider incorporating calming colors and decor to make your practice space inviting and relaxing. Soft blues, greens, and earthy tones can create a serene environment. Adding elements of nature, like plants or flowers, can enhance the sense of tranquility. I often find that a few well-placed plants can make a room feel more alive and peaceful. Playing soft, ambient music can also help set the mood. Choose tracks with gentle melodies or nature sounds that help you relax and focus. Having a playlist ready can make it easier to transition into your practice, creating a ritual that signals it's time to unwind.

Consistency is key to reaping the benefits of somatic exercises. Having a regular practice space helps build a routine. Designating a specific area for your exercises becomes a sacred space that encourages discipline and consistency. A consistent practice schedule is equally important. Whether it's first thing in the morning, during a lunch break, or before bed, find a time that works best for you and stick to it. Personalizing your space can also boost motivation. Add items that inspire you, such as motivational quotes, a vision board, or even family photos. These personal touches make the space yours, fostering a deeper connection to your practice.

COMMON MISCONCEPTIONS DEBUNKED

One of the most common misconceptions I encounter about somatic exercises is that they are solely for physical benefits. This belief couldn't be further from the truth. While it's true that somatic exercises can improve flexibility, posture, and alleviate pain, their impact extends far beyond the physical realm. These practices offer profound mental and emotional benefits. By engaging in mindful movement, you can reduce stress, manage anxiety, and build emotional resilience. The holistic nature of somatic exercises lies in their ability to integrate the mind and body, creating harmony and balance that permeates all aspects of life.

I've seen people experience holistic improvements in ways they never expected. For instance, a friend once told me how somatic exercises not only helped her with chronic shoulder pain but also improved her emotional well-being. She felt more grounded, less anxious, and better equipped to handle the stresses of daily life. These exercises provide a space for introspection and self-awareness, allowing you to tune into your emotions and understand them better. This emotional clarity can lead to healthier relationships, more effective stress management, and a greater sense of inner peace.

Another misconception is that somatic exercises are too simple to be effective. The beauty of these practices lies in their simplicity, but don't let that fool you into thinking they lack depth or effectiveness. Simple movements often mask complex processes that work on a neuromuscular level. For example, a basic exercise like lying on your back and slowly lifting your pelvis may seem straightforward. However, it involves intricate neuromuscular coordination and sensory awareness. These subtle movements can release deeply held tension and retrain your brain to move more efficiently.

Scientific research backs the effectiveness of these seemingly simple exercises. Studies have shown that somatic practices can significantly improve pain management, stress reduction, and emotional resilience. The science of neuroplasticity, the brain's ability to reorganize itself, supports the idea that mindful movement can create lasting changes in how we move and feel. By engaging in these exercises regularly, you're not just going through the motions; you're actively reshaping your brain and body for the better.

People often confuse somatic exercises with yoga or Pilates, but they differ fundamentally. While yoga and Pilates also emphasize body awareness and control, somatic exercises have a unique focus on sensory awareness and neuromuscular re-education. In yoga, you might hold a pose and focus on your breath. In somatic exercises, the emphasis is on the sensation of the movement itself, continually adjusting and exploring to find ease and comfort. This approach makes somatic exercises more adaptable and accessible, especially for those who might find traditional forms of exercise challenging or intimidating.

Lastly, let's dispel the notion that somatic exercises require prior experience or a certain fitness level. These exercises are designed to be beginner-friendly, with step-by-step guidance that makes them accessible to everyone. You don't need special skills or prior knowledge to benefit from somatic practices. I've worked with people of all ages and fitness levels, from teenagers to seniors, and the feedback is consistently positive. One of my students, who had never engaged in any form of exercise before, found somatic exercises to be a revelation. She appreciated the gentle, non-intimidating approach and quickly noticed improvements in her physical comfort and emotional well-being.

To wrap up, somatic exercises offer a holistic approach to well-being that addresses both the body and mind. They are simple yet profound, scientifically backed, and suitable for anyone, regardless of prior experience. As you continue to explore and practice these exercises, you'll find that they offer a path to a more balanced, joyful, and resilient life.

2

GETTING STARTED

I remember the first time I decided to commit to somatic exercises. It was a chilly morning, and I had just woken up feeling unusually stiff and mentally drained. The thought of diving into a new routine was daunting, yet something inside me knew that this practice could offer the relief I desperately needed. I took a deep breath, laid out my mat, and intended to simply explore and listen to my body. That small commitment changed everything for me and can for you too.

HOW TO BEGIN: A STEP-BY-STEP GUIDE

Preparation is key when starting any new practice, and somatic exercises are no exception. Before you dive in, take a moment to set your intentions. Ask yourself why you are embarking on this journey. Is it to relieve stress, manage pain, or build emotional resilience? Whatever your reasons, acknowledging them will give your practice purpose and direction. Once your intentions are clear, choose a consistent time and place for your exercises. Consistency helps build a routine, turning your practice into a habit. Whether it's first thing in the morning, during a lunch break, or before bed, find a time that works best for you and stick to it. Also, gather any necessary equipment, such as a comfortable mat and loose clothing, to ensure you have everything you need to get started.

With your preparations in place, it's time to take the first steps. Begin with simple, foundational exercises that are easy to follow. These initial movements will help you get accustomed to the practice without overwhelming you. For example, start with basic stretches and gentle movements focusing on releasing tension and improving body awareness. As you grow more comfortable, gradually increase the complexity of the exercises. This gradual progression allows your body to adapt and prevents the risk of injury. Always listen to your body; it will guide you. If an exercise feels too intense, scale it back. If you feel comfortable, try pushing a little further. The key is to find a balance that works for you.

Common beginner mistakes can hinder your progress but are easily avoidable with some awareness. One of the most common pitfalls is overexerting in the initial sessions. It's natural to feel enthusiastic and want to push yourself, but somatic exercises are about mindful, gentle movements. Overexertion can lead to strain and discomfort, which can discourage you from continuing. Another mistake is ignoring pain signals. Pain is your body's way of telling you something isn't right. If you experience pain during an exercise, stop immediately and reassess your form. Pain should never be a part of your practice; instead, aim for a feeling of gentle stretching and release.

Staying motivated in the early stages can be challenging, but there are several strategies you can employ. Start by setting small, achievable goals. Rather than aiming for an hour-long session, begin with just 10 minutes a day. Small goals are easier to achieve and can build a sense of accomplishment. Keeping a progress journal can also be incredibly motivating. Document your experiences, noting any improvements in flexibility, stress levels, or overall well-being. This record will serve as a tangible reminder of your progress. Celebrating small victories is another great way to stay motivated. Each time you complete a session or notice an improvement, take a moment to acknowledge and celebrate your achievement. This positive reinforcement will keep you engaged and excited about your practice. Need a progress tracker or a place to reflect on your practice? Download the free workbook in the Bonus Material section for helpful tools and resources.

Setting clear intentions, choosing a consistent time and place, and gathering the necessary equipment pave the way for a successful start. Begin with simple exercises, gradually increase complexity, and always listen to your body to avoid common pitfalls like overexertion and ignoring pain signals. Stay motivated by setting small goals, keeping a progress journal, and celebrating your victories, no matter how small they may seem.

BASIC PRINCIPLES OF BODY AWARENESS

Body awareness is a fundamental aspect of somatic exercises, rooted in the concept of proprioception. Proprioception is your body's ability to sense its position and movement in space. It allows you to touch your nose with your eyes closed or navigate a dark room without tripping. This sense is crucial for movement efficiency, as it helps you coordinate your actions and maintain balance. When you enhance body awareness, you better understand how your body moves and functions, leading to more controlled and intentional movements. This awareness is the cornerstone of somatic exercises, guiding you to move in mindful ways that are beneficial to your overall well-being.

To improve body awareness, start with mindful movement practices. These practices involve paying close attention to the sensations in your body as you move. For example, when you stretch your arms overhead, notice how your shoulders feel, the lengthening of your torso, and the expansion of your ribcage. This focused attention helps you become more attuned to your body's signals, allowing you to adjust your movements for greater ease and comfort. Sensory scanning is another effective technique. This practice involves mentally scanning your body from head to toe and observing any areas of tension or discomfort. By regularly performing sensory scans, you can identify and address issues before they become problematic.

The benefits of heightened body awareness are numerous. Improved coordination and balance are among the most immediate advantages. You're less likely to stumble or make awkward, inefficient movements when you're more aware of your body's position and movements. This improvement not only enhances your performance in physical activities but also reduces the risk of injury in daily life. Additionally, heightened body awareness can lead to better posture and alignment. Regularly tuning into your body's signals can correct imbalances and adopt more ergonomic positions, reducing strain on your muscles and joints.

Incorporating specific exercises can help you practice and enhance body awareness. Simple standing balance exercises are a great place to start. Stand on one leg, holding the position for 30 seconds to a minute, then switch to the other leg. Notice how your body compensates to maintain balance. Are you swaying or tensing certain muscles? Use this information to make small adjustments, improving your stability. Mindful walking is another excellent exercise. As you walk, pay attention to the sensation of your feet touching the ground, the movement of your legs, and the rhythm of your breath. This practice transforms an everyday activity into an opportunity for mindfulness and body awareness.

Integrating these techniques and exercises into your routine can cultivate a deeper connection with your body. This connection empowers you to move with greater intention and efficiency, enhancing your overall quality of life. As you continue to practice, you'll find that this heightened awareness extends beyond your exercise sessions, influencing how you carry yourself throughout the day. This newfound body awareness will serve as a foundation for more advanced somatic practices, enabling you to explore and enjoy the full range of benefits somatic exercises offer.

WARMING UP AND STRETCHING TECHNIQUES FOR BEGINNERS

When beginning somatic exercises, it's essential to recognize the significance of warming up and stretching. These foundational steps prepare your body for movement, improve flexibility, and reduce the risk of injury. Think of it as setting the stage for a productive session, where your muscles become pliable, responsive, and ready for the upcoming exercises. Whether new to somatic exercises or looking to enhance your practice, a well-rounded warm-up and stretching routine can make all the difference.

WARM-UP ROUTINES: PREPARING YOUR BODY

Effective warm-up exercises don't need to be complicated. Simple joint rotations are a great place to start. Begin with your neck, gently rotating it in a circular motion to release tension. Move on to shoulder rolls, rolling them forward and backward to open up your chest and upper back. Your wrists and ankles will also benefit from gentle rotations to improve flexibility and reduce stiffness. Light cardio movements, such as marching in place or gentle jogging, elevate your heart rate and increase blood flow, helping your entire body feel more prepared for the workout.

1. Neck Rotations

- **Instructions**: Perform five slow circles with your neck in each direction.
- **Cue**: Keep your shoulders relaxed and breathe deeply as you rotate your neck.

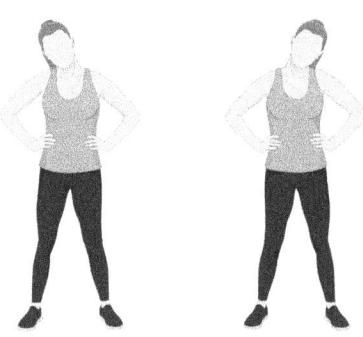

2. Shoulder Rolls

- **Instructions**: Roll your shoulders ten times forward, then ten times backward.
- **Cue**: Keep your back straight and make the movement smooth and controlled.

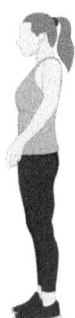 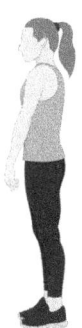

3. Arm Circles

- **Instructions**: Extend your arms to your sides and make small circles, gradually increasing the size for 30 seconds.
- **Cue**: Keep your arms straight but relaxed, and move in a controlled manner.

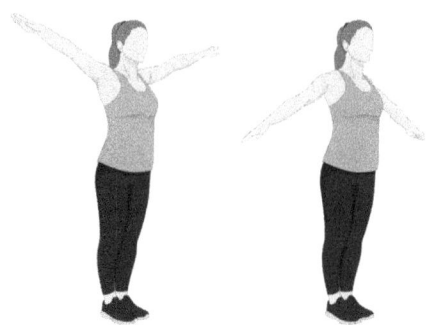

4. Wrist Rotations

- **Instructions**: Rotate each wrist ten times in both directions.
- **Cue**: Keep your arms relaxed and focus on smooth wrist movement.

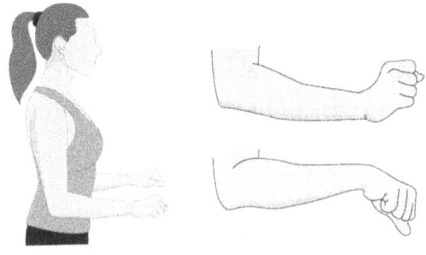

5. Torso Twists

- **Instructions**: With your feet planted, gently twist your upper body from side to side.
- **Cue**: Keep your hips still and let the twist come from your waist. Move slowly and breathe deeply.

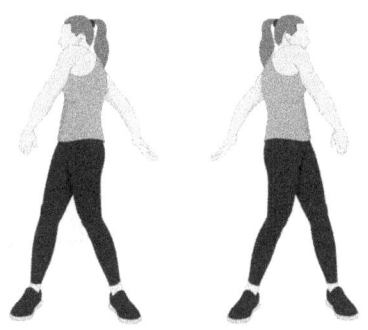

6. Ankle Rotations

- **Instructions**: Rotate each ankle in circles, ten times in each direction.
- **Cue**: Keep your leg relaxed and focus on making smooth, controlled circles with your ankle.

36 | SOMATIC EXERCISES FOR BEGINNERS

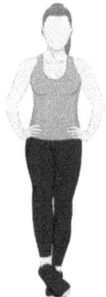 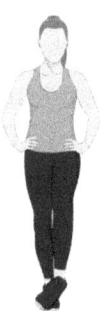

7. **March in Place**

- **Instructions**: Lightly march or jog in place for one minute to increase your heart rate.
- **Cue**: Keep your knees slightly lifted, move at a comfortable pace, and maintain steady breathing.

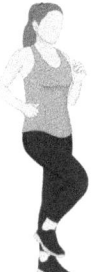 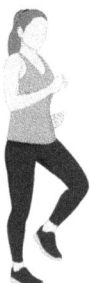

Quick Tip: For each exercise, listen to your body and adjust the intensity as needed. These movements should feel comfortable, not forced. Focus on your breathing throughout the warm-up to prepare both your body and mind.

Here's a structured warm-up routine:

- **Neck rotations:** Perform five circles in each direction.
- **Shoulder rolls:** Roll your shoulders ten times forward, then ten times backward.
- **Arm circles:** Extend your arms to your sides and make small circles, gradually increasing their size for 30 seconds.
- **Wrist rotations:** Rotate each wrist ten times in both directions.
- **Torso twists:** With your feet planted, gently twist your upper body from side to side.
- **Ankle rotations:** Rotate each ankle in circles, ten times in each direction.
- **March in place:** Lightly march or jog in place for one minute to increase your heart rate.

Customizing your warm-up is vital to address your unique needs. If you're a beginner, start with shorter durations and fewer repetitions, gradually increasing as you become more comfortable. Focus more on areas of tension or stiffness. For example, if your shoulders often feel tight, spend extra time on shoulder rolls. The key is to listen to your body and adjust your routine to suit how you're feeling on any given day.

Simple Stretching Techniques: Enhancing Flexibility

Stretching is an essential part of somatic exercises, playing a pivotal role in improving flexibility, muscle health, and injury prevention. Regular stretching allows your body to move more freely and efficiently, countering the negative effects of a sedentary lifestyle or repetitive movements. When you stretch, you increase blood flow to your muscles, helping them function better and recover faster.

To get the most out of your stretches, aim to hold each one for 20-30 seconds. This gives your muscles time to relax and lengthen. Breathing is also essential—inhale deeply as you prepare to stretch, and exhale slowly as you move into the stretch. This not only helps you get deeper into the stretch but also promotes relaxation.

Here are some beginner-friendly stretches that target key muscle groups:

1. Neck Stretch

- **Instructions**: Gently tilt your head to one side, bringing your ear toward your shoulder. Hold for 20-30 seconds, then switch sides.
- **Cue**: Keep your shoulders relaxed and breathe deeply as you stretch your neck.

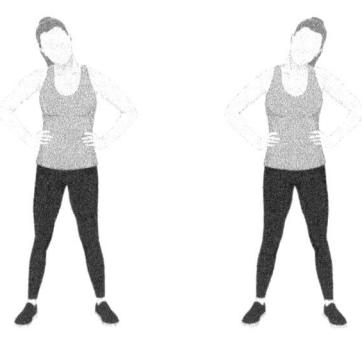

2. Shoulder Rolls

- **Instructions**: Roll your shoulders forward and backward to release tension. Repeat 10 times in each direction.
- **Cue**: Keep your back straight and move in a smooth, controlled motion.

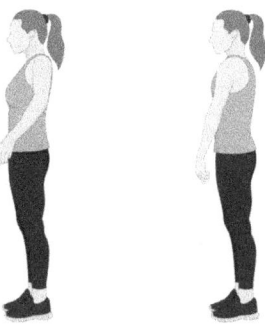

3. Seated Forward Fold

- **Instructions**: Sit on the floor with your legs extended in front of you and gently reach toward your toes, keeping your back straight. This stretches your hamstrings and lower back.
- **Cue**: Avoid rounding your back. Focus on hinging from your hips as you reach forward.

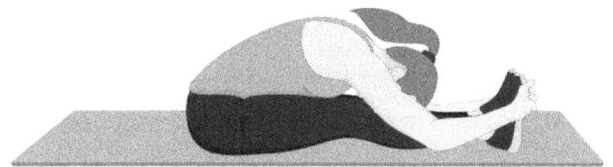

4. Butterfly Stretch

- **Instructions**: Sit with the soles of your feet touching and your knees bent outward. Gently press your knees toward the floor with your elbows, holding for 20-30 seconds to open your hips.
- **Cue**: Keep your back straight and gently apply pressure with your elbows to deepen the stretch.

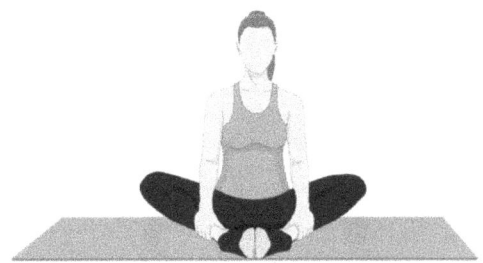

Quick Tip:

For each stretch, focus on deep breathing to help your muscles relax. Never force a stretch—only go as far as is comfortable and gradually work toward deeper flexibility over time.

- **Neck stretch:** Gently tilt your head to one side, bringing your ear toward your shoulder. Hold for 20-30 seconds, then switch sides.
- **Shoulder rolls:** Roll your shoulders forward and backward to release tension.
- **Seated forward fold:** Sit on the floor with your legs extended and gently reach toward your toes, keeping your back straight. This stretches your hamstrings and lower back.

- **Butterfly stretch:** Sit with the soles of your feet touching and your knees bent outward. Gently press your knees toward the floor with your elbows, holding for 20-30 seconds to open your hips.

To create a structured stretching routine:

- Begin with **neck and shoulder stretches** to release upper body tension.
- Move on to **lower back and hamstring stretches** to loosen stiff areas in your legs and back.
- Finish with **hip and thigh stretches** to open your hips and improve flexibility.

Aim to spend 5-10 minutes on this routine each day, holding each stretch for 20-30 seconds and repeating as needed. You can integrate these stretches into your daily life, whether it's in the morning to wake up your body or in the evening to unwind before bed. Consistent stretching will improve your flexibility and muscle health and enhance your overall sense of well-being.

By incorporating both warm-up and stretching techniques into your somatic exercise routine, you'll set yourself up for success. These foundational practices prepare your body, improve flexibility, and ensure you get the most out of your exercise sessions, leaving you feeling more relaxed, agile, and ready to take on the day.

HOW TO PERFORM A BODY SCAN MEDITATION

The first time I attempted a body scan meditation, I was skeptical. I had heard about its benefits—how it could help with relaxation and enhance body awareness—but I wasn't sure it would work for me. I found a quiet spot, laid down on my mat, and decided to give it a try. To my surprise, the experience was transformative. Body scan meditation is a mindfulness practice where you focus sequentially on different parts of your body, observing sensations without judgment. This practice helps you tune into your body's needs and promotes deep relaxation. By paying attention to each area, you can identify and release tension, improving overall body awareness.

Begin by finding a comfortable position. You can lie down on your back with your legs extended and arms resting at your sides, palms facing up. If lying down is uncomfortable, sit in a chair with your feet flat on the floor and your hands resting on your thighs. Close your eyes and take a few deep breaths, settling into the present moment. Start by focusing on your toes. Notice any sensations—tingling, warmth, coolness, or even numbness. Without trying to change anything, just observe. Slowly move your attention up to your feet, ankles, calves, and so on until you reach the top of your head. Take your time with each area, allowing yourself to fully experience whatever sensations arise.

Maintaining focus during a body scan meditation can be challenging, especially for beginners. It's natural for your mind to wander. When this happens, gently bring your attention back to the part of the body you were focusing on. Use your breath as an anchor, taking slow, deep breaths to help maintain your focus. Each time you inhale, imagine sending your breath to the area you're focusing on, and with each exhale, imagine releasing any tension. This technique not only helps you stay present but also enhances the relaxation effect of the practice.

Beginners often face common challenges when starting body scan meditation. Distractions are a big one. It's easy to get pulled away by external noises or internal thoughts. When this happens, acknowledge the distraction without judgment and gently bring your focus back to your body. Another challenge is staying patient with the process. It's normal to feel restless or impatient, especially if you're not used to sitting still. Remind yourself that it's okay to feel this way and that you're building your ability to stay present every time you practice. Start with shorter sessions, gradually increasing the duration as you become more comfortable.

Using guided meditations can be particularly helpful for beginners. Many apps and audio resources offer guided body scan meditations. Some popular ones include Headspace, Calm, and Insight Timer. These guided sessions provide verbal instructions, making it easier to stay focused and follow along. The gentle voice of a guide can also be soothing, helping you relax more deeply. As you become more familiar with the practice, you may prefer unguided sessions, but guided meditations are a great way to get started.

The experience of a body scan meditation can be profoundly calming and insightful. It's a simple yet powerful practice that helps you connect more deeply with your body and mind. By regularly incorporating body scan meditation into your routine, you'll become more attuned to your body's signals, better able to manage stress, and more skilled at releasing tension. This practice enhances your somatic exercises and contributes to your overall well-being.

CUSTOMIZING YOUR EXERCISE PLAN: TIPS AND TRICKS

When I began my journey with somatic exercises, I quickly realized that a one-size-fits-all approach wouldn't work. Each of us has unique needs, goals, and limitations. That's why tailoring your somatic exercise plan is so crucial. Recognizing your personal goals is the first step. Are you looking to relieve chronic pain, reduce stress, or improve overall flexibility? Identifying your primary objective helps you focus your efforts and choose exercises that align with your intentions. Adapting exercises to your fitness level is equally important. If you're just starting out, you'll want to begin with gentler movements before progressing to more challenging ones. On the other hand, if you're more experienced, you can incorporate advanced techniques to keep yourself engaged.

Addressing specific pain points and stress areas can make your practice more effective. For instance, if you suffer from lower back pain, you'll want to include exercises that strengthen your core and improve your posture. If stress is your main concern, integrating breathwork and relaxation techniques will be beneficial. By focusing on your unique needs, you can create a plan that meets your goals and enhances your overall well-being.

To personalize your somatic exercise plan:

1. Start by assessing your needs and limitations.
2. Take note of any areas of discomfort or stiffness, and consider your fitness level.
3. Choose exercises that resonate with you.

For example, if you enjoy gentle stretching, incorporate more of those movements into your routine. Adjust the intensity and duration based on your progress. If you find a particular exercise too challenging, modify it or reduce the time you spend on it. Conversely, if an exercise feels too easy, try increasing the intensity or adding a new element to keep it challenging.

Customizing your somatic exercise plan can transform your practice, making it more enjoyable, effective, and sustainable. By recognizing your personal goals, adapting exercises to your fitness level, and addressing specific pain points and stress areas, you create a plan that truly works for you. This personalized approach increases motivation and adherence, enhances the relevance and effectiveness of your practice, and provides a deeper sense of satisfaction.

3

STRESS AND ANXIETY RELIEF

I remember one particularly chaotic day when everything seemed to be spiraling out of control. My to-do list was a mile long, my phone wouldn't stop ringing, and I felt like I was on the verge of a breakdown. In the midst of this chaos, I took a moment to sit down, close my eyes, and focus on my breath. Almost immediately, I felt a sense of calm wash over me. This simple act of mindful breathing became my sanctuary, a way to find peace amidst the storm. It's incredible how something as basic as breathing can profoundly impact our mental state.

BREATHING TECHNIQUES FOR INSTANT CALM

Importance of Breathwork in Somatic Exercises

The role of breathwork in somatic exercises is pivotal. Breath is not just a function of life but a powerful tool that can significantly enhance your practice. Think about the last time you felt stressed or anxious. Chances are, your breathing became shallow and rapid. This is your body's natural response to stress, but it also means that controlling your breath can help manage stress. In somatic exercises, breath and movement are deeply intertwined. Coordinating your breath with your movements not only makes the exercises more effective but also helps you tune into your body more deeply. Focusing on your breath anchors yourself in the present moment, making it easier to release tension and stress.

The breath serves as a tool for relaxation, guiding your body into a state of calm. When you take slow, deep breaths, you activate the parasympathetic nervous system, which is responsible for the body's rest and digestion functions. This activation counteracts the stress response, lowering your heart rate and relaxing your muscles. The beauty of breathwork lies in its simplicity and accessibility. You don't need special equipment or a specific setting to practice it. Whether at home, at work, or even in a crowded place, you can always return to your breath to find a moment of calm.

Proper breathwork offers numerous physiological benefits. Improved oxygenation is one of the most immediate effects. When you breathe deeply and fully, you increase the amount of oxygen that reaches your cells, enhancing overall vitality. This improved oxygenation also supports better circulation, ensuring that your muscles receive the nutrients they need to function optimally. Enhanced muscle relaxation is another significant benefit. As you practice deep breathing, your muscles naturally begin to release tension, promoting a sense of ease and relaxation throughout your body.

One of the most effective breathing techniques for calming the mind is diaphragmatic breathing. This method focuses on deep, belly-centered breaths, engaging your diaphragm fully.

Diaphragmatic breathing:

1. Start by sitting or lying down in a comfortable position.
2. Place one hand on your chest and the other on your belly.
3. Inhale deeply through your nose, letting your belly rise as you fill your lungs with air. Your chest should remain relatively still.
4. Exhale slowly through your mouth, feeling your belly fall.

This technique ensures that you are using your diaphragm to its full capacity, promoting deeper, more efficient breaths. Practicing this for just a few minutes can help reduce stress and bring a sense of peace.

Another effective technique is box breathing, which involves a structured pattern of inhaling, holding the breath, exhaling, and holding again, each for a count of four. This method helps regulate your breath and can be particularly useful in high-stress situations.

Box Breathing Technique:

- Sit comfortably with your back straight and your feet flat on the floor.
- Inhale deeply through your nose for a count of four, feeling your lungs fill with air.
- Hold your breath for another count of four.
- Exhale slowly through your mouth for a count of four, and then hold your breath again for a final count of four.
- Repeat this cycle for several minutes, allowing your breath to become a steady rhythm.

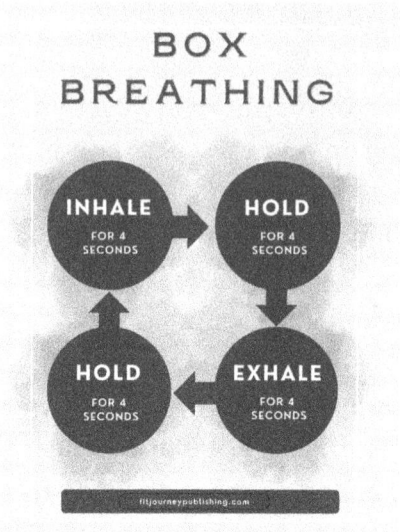

This technique calms your mind and trains you to maintain control over your breathing, even in stressful moments.

Let's put these techniques into practice with a guided session. Find a quiet space where you won't be disturbed. Sit or lie down comfortably, and close your eyes. Begin with diaphragmatic breathing: inhale deeply through your nose, letting your belly rise, and exhale slowly through your mouth, letting your belly fall. Continue this for two minutes, focusing on the rise and fall of your belly. Now, transition to box breathing. Inhale through your nose for a count of four, hold for four, exhale for four, and hold again for four. Continue this pattern for three minutes. As you breathe, imagine each breath bringing in calm and each exhale releasing tension. After five minutes, gently open your eyes and take a moment to notice how you feel. This short practice can be a powerful way to reset and find calm amidst stress.

STRESS AND ANXIETY RELIEF | 51

4-7-8 Breathing Technique

Another effective exercise is the 4-7-8 technique.

- **Sit comfortably** and close your eyes
- **Inhale** gently through your nose for a count of four, feeling your lungs expand.
- **Hold your breath** for a count of seven, allowing the air to settle in your lungs.
- **Exhale completely** through your mouth for a count of eight, focusing on releasing any tension as you breathe out.
- **Repeat this cycle four times**, letting your body relax more deeply with each breath.

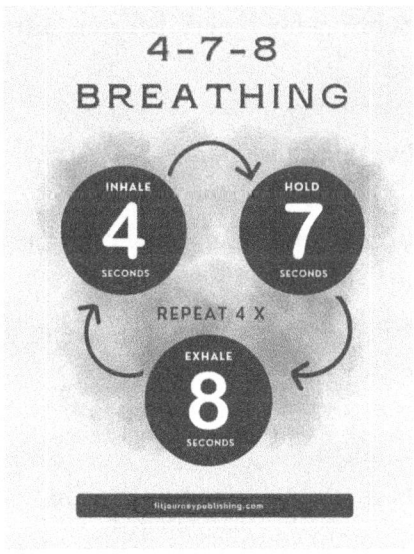

HEART-CENTERED BREATHING FOR COMPASSION

Heart-centered breathing is a powerful technique that focuses on directing your breath to your heart, fostering feelings of compassion and empathy. This practice involves visualizing your breath as if it's flowing in and out of your heart, creating a warm, nurturing sensation. Connecting your breath with your heart center can cultivate a deeper sense of emotional well-being and relational harmony. The benefits of this practice are profound. Heart-centered breathing can increase your feelings of empathy, allowing you to connect more deeply with others. It also enhances your ability to manage difficult emotions, providing a sense of inner peace and resilience. As you breathe through your heart, you may find that your emotional responses become more balanced, and your interactions with others become more compassionate and understanding.

Heart-Centered Breathing Technique

- **Find a quiet, comfortable space** where you can relax without disturbance.
- **Sit or lie down** in a relaxed position, and place one hand gently over your heart.
- **Close your eyes** and take a few deep breaths to settle into the present moment.
- **Inhale deeply** through your nose, imagining the breath flowing directly into your heart, feeling warmth and compassion as your chest expands.
- **Hold the breath** for a moment, savoring the feeling of calm in your heart.
- **Exhale slowly** through your mouth, visualizing warmth and kindness spreading throughout your body and beyond.

- **Continue this pattern**—inhaling deeply, holding briefly, and exhaling slowly—focusing on the sensation of your hand on your heart as a grounding anchor.

This heart-centered breathing practice can help cultivate compassion, calm, and emotional resilience, making it a perfect addition to your daily routine.

The emotional and relational benefits of heart-centered breathing are significant. By regularly practicing this technique, you can increase your feelings of empathy and connectedness with others. This deeper sense of connection can improve your relationships, fostering greater understanding and compassion. Heart-centered breathing also enhances your emotional resilience, making it easier to navigate challenging situations with grace and composure. As you become more adept at this practice, you'll find that it promotes overall emotional well-being, helping you maintain a balanced and peaceful state of mind.

These breathwork practices are simple yet powerful tools that can significantly enhance your somatic exercise routine. They help you connect more deeply with your body, promote relaxation, and improve overall physical and mental well-being. As you continue to explore these techniques, you'll find that they become an integral part of your practice, offering immediate relief and long-term benefits.

MINDFULNESS PRACTICES FOR DAILY STRESS

Mindfulness is a practice that has transformed my own approach to managing daily stress. At its core, mindfulness is about present-moment awareness—being fully engaged with whatever you're doing right now. This might sound simple, but in our fast-paced lives, it can be surprisingly challenging. The benefits of mindfulness are both psychological and physiological. When you focus on the present, you reduce the constant mental chatter that fuels stress and anxiety. This mental clarity can lower blood pressure, improve sleep, and even enhance your overall mood.

One of the simplest ways to practice mindfulness is through mindful breathing, such as diaphragmatic breathing, box breathing, or heart centered breathing. As you breathe, notice the sensation of the air entering and leaving your body. If your mind starts to wander, gently bring your focus back to your breath. This practice can be done anywhere and only takes a few minutes, making it an excellent tool for managing stress during a busy day.

Additionally, incorporating mindful movement into your routine can also be incredibly beneficial. Slow, deliberate movements like mindful walking can help ground you in the present moment. As you walk, pay attention to the sensation of your feet touching the ground, the rhythm of your steps, and the movement of your body. Another effective practice is a body scan with movement. Begin at your feet and slowly move your attention up through your body, noticing any areas of tension or discomfort. As you identify these areas, gently stretch or move them to release the tension. This combination of mindfulness and movement can make your practice more dynamic and engaging.

Mindfulness can be seamlessly integrated into everyday activities, turning routine tasks into moments of calm and focus. For instance, try practicing mindful eating. As you eat, pay close attention to the flavors, textures, and aromas of your food. Chew slowly and savor each bite, fully immersing yourself in the experience. This enhances your enjoyment of the meal and helps you become more aware of your body's hunger and fullness signals. Another practical tip is to incorporate mindfulness into routine tasks like brushing your teeth. Focus on the sensation of the toothbrush against your teeth, the taste of the toothpaste, and the sound of the bristles. These small moments of mindfulness can accumulate, significantly reducing your overall stress levels.

GUIDED IMAGERY: VISUALIZING PEACE AND CALM

One of the most transformative tools I've discovered for relaxation is guided imagery. This technique uses visualization to promote relaxation and reduce stress by engaging your imagination. Imagine your mind as a canvas and your thoughts as the paintbrush. By creating vivid mental images, you can evoke a sense of calm and strengthen your mind-body connection. Guided imagery allows you to mentally transport yourself to a peaceful setting, effectively reducing stress and promoting a sense of well-being.

To practice guided imagery, start by choosing a peaceful scene or setting that makes you feel relaxed and happy. This could be a serene beach, a lush forest, or even a cozy room with a fireplace. The key is to select a place where you feel safe and at ease. Close your eyes and begin to visualize this scene in as much detail as possible. Engage all your senses in the visualization. Imagine the sound of waves crashing on the shore, the scent of pine trees, or the warmth of the fire. The more detailed and immersive your visualization, the more effective it will be.

For a successful guided imagery practice, consider these tips. Practicing in a quiet, comfortable space is essential to minimize distractions. Using guided audio recordings can also be incredibly helpful, especially if you're new to the practice. These recordings provide gentle instructions and soothing sounds that can enhance your focus and relaxation. Combining guided imagery with deep breathing can further amplify its calming effects. As you visualize your peaceful scene, take slow, deep breaths, allowing the imagery and breath to work together to promote relaxation.

The benefits of guided imagery are immediate and profound. As you immerse yourself in the visualization, you'll likely feel a sense of calm and relaxation wash over you. This practice can also improve your emotional well-being by providing a mental escape from daily stresses. Additionally, guided imagery enhances mental clarity and focus, making it easier to manage tasks and challenges with a clear, calm mind. By regularly practicing guided imagery, you can create a mental sanctuary that you can return to whenever you need a break from the chaos of daily life.

GROUNDING EXERCISES TO STAY PRESENT

Grounding is a powerful technique that helps you stay present and manage anxiety. At its core, grounding connects you to the present moment, making it an integral part of mindfulness. When you're grounded, you're anchored in the here and now, which can significantly reduce anxiety and intrusive thoughts. This practice helps break the cycle of worry by shifting your focus to what's happening right now, rather than what might happen in the future or what has happened in the past.

5-4-3-2-1 Grounding Technique

- Take a deep breath and look around you.
- **Identify five things you can see**, such as a picture on the wall, a tree outside, or any objects in your environment.
- **Focus on four things you can touch**, like the texture of your clothes, the feeling of your chair, or anything within reach.
- **Listen for three sounds**, whether it's the hum of an appliance, birds chirping, or any other noises in your surroundings.

- **Identify two things you can smell**, such as a candle, your surroundings, or the fresh air.
- **Notice one thing you can taste**, even if it's just the lingering taste of your last meal or a sip of water.

By engaging all your senses, this technique helps ground you in the present moment, making it easier to manage anxiety and reconnect with your surroundings.

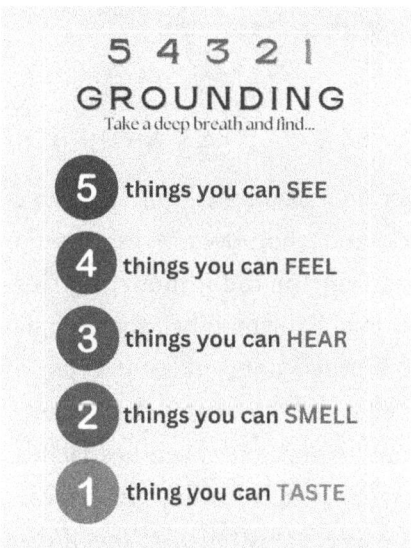

Physical grounding exercises can also be incredibly effective and can be done almost anywhere. Walking barefoot is a simple yet powerful way to ground yourself. Feel the texture of the ground beneath your feet, whether it's grass, sand, or even your living room floor. This physical connection to the earth can be incredibly calming. Another technique involves using pressure points. Press your hands together firmly and focus on the sensation of the pressure. This tactile experience can help anchor you to the present, providing a quick way to reduce anxiety.

Grounding exercises can be seamlessly integrated into your daily life. For example, if you find yourself feeling anxious during a meeting, you can discreetly use the 5-4-3-2-1 technique to calm your mind. Or, if you're feeling overwhelmed at home, take a few minutes to walk barefoot outside and reconnect with nature. I remember a particularly stressful day when I felt overwhelmed by a multitude of tasks. I stepped outside, took off my shoes, and walked slowly on the grass. The cool, soft sensation under my feet brought an immediate sense of calm, helping me reset and approach my tasks with a clearer mind.

TENSION RELEASE FOR NECK AND SHOULDERS

Stress has a sneaky way of manifesting itself in our bodies, particularly in the neck and shoulders. When you're under pressure, your body enters a fight-or-flight mode, causing muscles to tense up as a protective mechanism. This physiological response often results in tight, painful knots, making even simple movements uncomfortable. The common symptoms include stiffness, limited range of motion, and sometimes even headaches. These areas bear the brunt of our stress, often leading to chronic discomfort if not addressed. To counteract this tension, specific exercises can work wonders.

This routine is designed to help release tension in your neck and shoulders, using simple stretches and self-massage techniques. Perform each exercise slowly and mindfully, focusing on your breath and how your body feels.

1. Side Neck Stretch

- **Instructions**: Sit or stand comfortably and gently tilt your head toward one shoulder, bringing your ear closer to it. Hold the stretch for 20-30 seconds, feeling the gentle pull along the side of your neck. Repeat on the other side.
- **Cue**: Keep your shoulders relaxed and focus on the stretch in your neck, not forcing it.

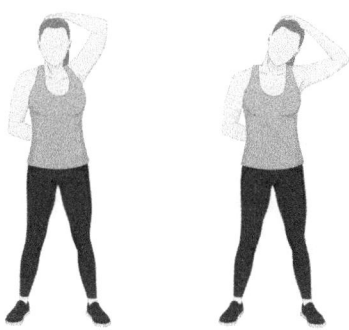

2. Shoulder Rolls

- **Instructions**: Sit or stand with your back straight and slowly roll your shoulders forward in a circular motion for about 15-20 seconds. Then reverse the direction and roll them backward for another 15-20 seconds.
- **Cue**: Keep the motion slow and controlled, and breathe deeply throughout the movement.

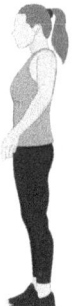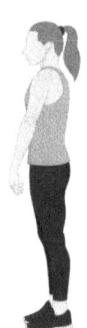

3. Shoulder Shrugs

- **Instructions**: Lift your shoulders toward your ears, hold for a few seconds, and then release. Repeat this movement 5-10 times to relieve tension.
- **Cue**: As you release your shoulders, exhale deeply and feel the tension melt away.

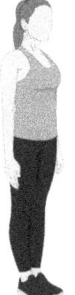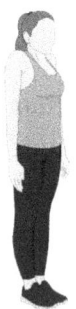

4. Self-Massage Techniques

- **A. Neck Massage**: Using your fingertips, gently massage the muscles at the base of your skull, working your way down the sides of your neck. Apply gentle pressure and use circular motions to release any tight spots.
  - **Cue**: Focus on areas that feel tight, using small, slow circular motions to ease tension.
- **B. Shoulder Blade Massage**: Reach across your body with one hand to the opposite shoulder blade. Use your fingers to knead the muscles there, applying pressure to release deep-seated tension.
  - **Cue**: Move slowly, applying as much pressure as feels comfortable to release tension in the muscles.

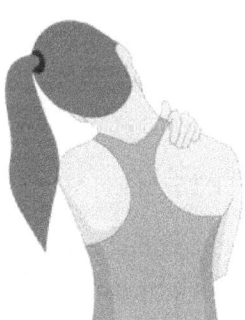 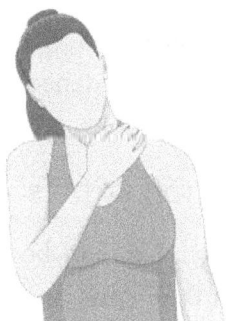

Quick Tip:

When performing these stretches and massages, remember to breathe deeply. Inhaling helps you focus, and exhaling allows you to relax into the stretch or massage.

A sample routine for tension relief for neck and shoulders could look like this:

1. **Side Neck Stretch** - hold on each side for 20- 30 seconds
2. **Shoulder Rolls** - 15-20 seconds in each direction
3. **Shoulder Shrugs** - Perform 10-15 times
4. **Self Massage - Neck and Shoulder Blade Area**

Aim to practice this routine daily, ideally in the morning or before bed, to maximize its benefits.

Incorporating a quick tension release routine into your daily practice can make a significant difference. This routine should take no more than five minutes and can be easily integrated into your morning or evening routine. You can even do it during a quick break at work to refresh and reset. By regularly practicing these exercises, you'll find that your neck and shoulders feel more relaxed and less burdened by the stresses of daily life.

SOMATIC EXERCISES FOR ANXIETY MANAGEMENT

Somatic exercises can be a lifeline when it comes to managing anxiety. At their core, these exercises work by calming the nervous system and enhancing body awareness, which helps mitigate anxiety. When you're anxious, your body is in a heightened state of alert, often triggering the fight-or-flight response. This leads to increased heart rate, shallow breathing, and muscle tension. Somatic exercises help counteract this by activating the parasympathetic nervous system, which promotes relaxation and reduces these physical symptoms. Moreover, by focusing on body awareness, you can better understand how anxiety manifests in your body and learn to release it more effectively.

One particularly effective somatic exercise for anxiety relief is progressive muscle relaxation.

Progressive Muscle Relaxation for Anxiety Relief

- **Find a comfortable position**, either sitting or lying down.
- **Close your eyes** and take a few deep breaths to center yourself.
- **Start with your feet**: Inhale as you tense the muscles in your toes, then exhale as you release the tension.
- **Move to your calves**: Tense the muscles as you inhale, and release as you exhale.
- **Progress to your thighs**, repeating the same tensing and releasing motion.
- **Focus on your abdomen**: Tense the muscles as you inhale, then release with your exhale.
- **Move to your chest**: Inhale, tense the muscles, and exhale, letting go of the tension.
- **Focus on your arms**, tensing your muscles as you inhale, and releasing as you exhale.
- **Finally, focus on your face**, tensing the muscles as you inhale and releasing them with your exhale.

As you work through each muscle group, **focus on the sensation of tension leaving your body**. This exercise reduces physical tension and provides a mental break from anxious thoughts, promoting a deep sense of relaxation.

Somatic Shaking for Anxiety Relief

- **Stand with your feet hip-width apart**, finding a stable and comfortable position.

- **Begin by shaking your hands**, letting the movements be loose and free.
- **Move to shaking your arms** and **shoulders**, allowing your body to move naturally.
- **Progress to shaking your entire body**, keeping the movement rhythmic and unrestricted.
- **Focus on releasing built-up tension** as you shake, letting go of stress and pent-up energy.
- **Continue for a few minutes**, letting your body move freely and naturally.
- **Regulate your breathing** as you shake, noticing the calming effect on your breath and heart rate.

Somatic shaking can be especially effective after a stressful day, helping to release tension, regulate your body, and promote a sense of calm.

Sensory integration plays a crucial role in managing anxiety through somatic exercises. Enhancing sensory perception allows you to ground yourself in the present moment and reduce anxious thoughts. Techniques to enhance sensory perception include focusing on touch, sight, and sound. For example, you can rub your hands together and notice the texture and warmth or focus on a soothing visual stimulus like a candle flame. Exercises involving sensory experiences can be incredibly grounding. One technique is to hold a textured object, like a stress ball, and focus on its texture and weight. Another is to listen to calming sounds, such as nature recordings or gentle music, which can help shift your focus away from anxiety.

Real-life examples highlight the effectiveness of these techniques. I recall my student Sarah who struggled with severe anxiety. She found progressive muscle relaxation to be a game-changer. By practicing it daily, she was able to significantly reduce her anxiety levels and improve her overall quality of life. A friend, Mark, found relief through somatic shaking. After incorporating it into his routine, he reported feeling more grounded and less overwhelmed by his anxiety. These personal stories underscore the transformative power of somatic exercises in managing anxiety.

CREATING A STRESS-RELIEF ROUTINE

One of the most transformative steps you can take for long-term stress management is establishing a consistent stress-relief routine. Habits are powerful, shaping our daily lives and influencing our well-being. By integrating stress-relief practices into your daily routine, you build habits that help sustain stress management over time. The psychological benefits are immense. Having a set routine provides a sense of stability and predictability, which can be incredibly comforting in our often chaotic lives. Knowing that you have dedicated time each day to focus on your well-being can alleviate anxiety and create a sense of control.

To create an effective stress-relief routine, start by choosing the right exercises that resonate with you. These could be simple somatic exercises, mindfulness practices, or even a combination of both. Next, set a regular practice time. Consistency is key, so find a time that fits seamlessly into your daily schedule. Make this time non-negotiable, whether first thing in the morning, during a lunch break, or before bed. This commitment to a regular schedule helps reinforce the habit, making it easier to stick to your routine in the long run.

Let's look at some sample routines tailored to different time availability and preferences. If you're short on time, a 5-minute quick relief routine can be incredibly effective. This could include a few minutes of diaphragmatic breathing followed by simple neck stretches. For those with a bit more time, a 20-minute comprehensive routine might be ideal. This could start with a body scan meditation, followed by some gentle somatic exercises like shoulder rolls, and end with a short period of guided imagery. If you prefer a relaxing end to your day, an evening wind-down routine can help you transition into sleep. This could involve gentle stretching, progressive muscle relaxation, and a few minutes of heart-centered breathing.

Maintaining consistency is crucial for the success of any routine. One effective strategy is setting reminders. Use your phone or a scheduling app to set daily alerts, reminding you to take your stress-relief break. Tracking your progress with a journal can also be motivating. Record how you feel before and after each session, noting any improvements in your stress levels or overall well-being. This tangible evidence of progress can keep you motivated. Don't forget, you can find printable resources, including detailed guides and trackers, in the **free workbook** located in the Bonus Material section at the front of this book. Finding a practice buddy can provide additional accountability. Whether it's a friend, family member, or even a co-worker, having someone to share the experience with can make it more enjoyable and help you stay committed.

4

PAIN MANAGEMENT

I remember waking up one morning with a relentless ache in my lower back. It was the kind of pain that made getting out of bed feel like climbing a mountain. After weeks of trying various remedies—painkillers and heat packs —I felt defeated. Nothing seemed to provide lasting relief. In addition to learning about somatic exercises for stress and anxiety, I had come across research on how these exercises were also beneficial for pain. To my surprise, the gentle, mindful movements started making a difference. The pain began to lessen, and I felt a sense of control returning. This experience opened my eyes to the potential of somatic exercises for managing chronic pain.

UNDERSTANDING CHRONIC PAIN AND SOMATIC EXERCISES

Chronic pain is a complex and often misunderstood condition. Unlike acute pain, which serves as an immediate warning signal that something is wrong in your body, chronic pain is persistent, lasting for months or even years. It is defined by the International

Association for the Study of Pain (IASP) as pain persisting or recurring for longer than three months. Chronic pain can manifest in various ways, including a dull ache, sharp stabbing sensations, or a burning feeling. Common causes include arthritis, nerve damage, or past injuries that never fully healed. Unlike acute pain, which usually resolves once the underlying issue is treated, chronic pain can continue even after the initial cause has been addressed.

One of the most challenging aspects of chronic pain is the cycle of pain and tension it creates. When you experience chronic pain, your body often responds by tensing up muscles around the painful area, trying to protect it. This muscle tension can, in turn, exacerbate the pain, creating a vicious cycle. Stress compounds this issue. When you're stressed, your body's natural response is to tighten muscles, which only adds to the existing tension. Over time, this cycle can become deeply ingrained, making it difficult to break without targeted intervention. The relationship between stress and muscle tension is well-documented, showing that managing stress is essential for alleviating chronic pain.

Somatic exercises play a crucial role in breaking this cycle of pain and tension. These exercises focus on body awareness, helping you become more attuned to your physical sensations and recognize areas of tension. Techniques like slow, deliberate movements and mindful breathing can help release muscle tension. For instance, the method of "pandiculation," developed by Thomas Hanna, involves slow, conscious movements that engage the nervous system in a relearning process, helping to release subconsciously held muscular contractions. This approach not only alleviates tension but also enhances flexibility and mobility, making it easier to move without pain. By regularly practicing somatic exercises, you can retrain your body to move efficiently and comfortably, reducing the impact of chronic pain.

Scientific evidence supports the effectiveness of somatic exercises in managing chronic pain. Research has shown that these practices can significantly reduce pain levels by addressing neuromuscular imbalances and promoting relaxation. A study published in the National Center for Biotechnology Information (NCBI) highlights the benefits of somatic practices for chronic pain management. The study found that these exercises enhance body awareness and self-regulation through movement, leading to reduced pain perception and improved quality of life. Additionally, experts like Sarah Warren, a Certified Clinical Somatic Educator, advocate for these techniques, emphasizing their ability to retrain the nervous system and alleviate pain. Clinical evidence also supports the positive impact of somatic exercises, with numerous testimonials from individuals who have experienced significant pain relief through these practices.

Understanding chronic pain and the role of somatic exercises in managing it can empower you to take control of your well-being. By breaking the cycle of pain and tension, improving body awareness, and incorporating scientifically-backed techniques, you can find lasting relief and enhance your overall quality of life.

EXERCISES FOR LOWER BACK PAIN RELIEF

Lower back pain is one of the most common ailments affecting people today. Statistics reveal that approximately 80% of adults experience lower back pain at some point in their lives. This prevalence is often due to a combination of factors such as poor posture, muscle imbalances, and sedentary lifestyles. For instance, sitting for prolonged periods can cause the muscles in your lower back to become tight and weak, leading to discomfort and pain. Additionally, conditions like herniated discs, sciatica, and muscle strain can all contribute to chronic lower back pain.

Understanding these common causes is the first step toward effective pain relief. Specific somatic exercises can make a significant difference in addressing lower back pain.

This routine focuses on releasing tension and building strength in your lower back and core. Each exercise should be performed with mindful breathing to maximize the benefits.

1. Pelvic Tilt

- **Instructions**: Start by lying on your back with your knees bent and feet flat on the floor. Slowly tilt your pelvis upward, flattening your lower back against the floor. Next, raise your pelvis off the floor, one vertebrae at a time until your hips line up with your shoulders and knees. Then slowly release by lowering your spine one vertebrae at the time, returning to the start position. Repeat 10-15 times, focusing on the sensations in your lower back and abdomen.
- **Cue**: Engage your core as you tilt your pelvis and focus on the subtle movement in your lower back.

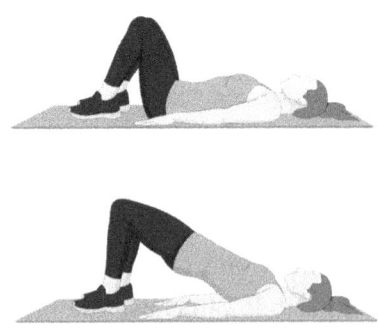

2. Cat-Cow Stretch

- **Instructions**: Begin on your hands and knees with your wrists aligned under your shoulders and your knees under your hips. Inhale as you arch your back, lifting your head and tailbone (Cow pose). Exhale as you round your back, tucking your chin and tailbone (Cat pose). Repeat the sequence 10-15 times, smoothly transitioning between the two poses.
- **Cue**: Synchronize your breath with the movement, deepening each stretch as you exhale.

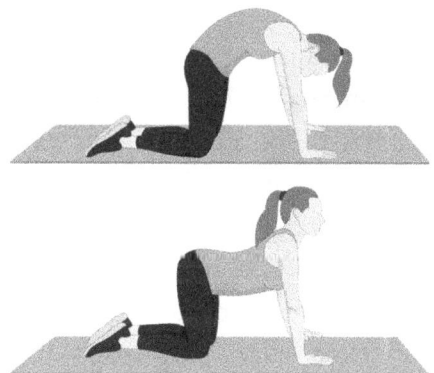

3. Child's Pose

- **Instructions**: Kneel on the floor, sit back on your heels, and stretch your arms forward, lowering your chest toward the floor. Hold this position for 30 seconds to 1 minute, breathing deeply and relaxing your entire body.
- **Cue**: Allow your hips to sink toward your heels and reach your arms forward to lengthen your spine.

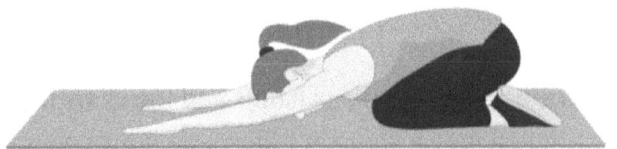

Quick Tip:

While performing these exercises, focus on using your breath to release any tension. The pelvic tilt will help activate your core, while the Cat-Cow and Child's Pose provide mobility and gentle release for your spine.

Each of these exercises offers unique benefits for alleviating lower back pain. Pelvic tilts help strengthen your core muscles, providing better support for your lower back and reducing strain. The Cat-Cow stretch improves spinal mobility, making it easier to move without discomfort. This exercise also helps release tension in the muscles along your spine. The Child's pose, on the other hand, provides a gentle stretch for your lower back and promotes relaxation. It helps lengthen the spine and release built-up tension, making it a great exercise to include in your routine, especially after a long day.

A sample routine for lower back pain relief could look like this:

2. **pelvic tilts** - Start with 10-15, focusing on controlled, slow movements.
3. **Cat-Cow stretch** -performing 10-15 repetitions, moving seamlessly between the poses.
4. **Child's pose** - holding the stretch for 30 seconds to 1 minute.

Aim to practice this routine daily, ideally in the morning or before bed, to maximize its benefits.

Integrating these exercises into your daily practice can help maintain flexibility and reduce lower back pain over time. Remember to listen to your body and adjust the exercises as needed, gradually increasing the duration or repetitions as you become more comfortable.

TECHNIQUES FOR ALLEVIATING NECK PAIN

Neck pain is a common issue that many of us face at some point. Often, it creeps up slowly, starting as a minor discomfort and gradually becoming a persistent ache. One of the leading causes is poor posture, especially in our modern world, where we spend countless hours hunched over computers and smartphones. This constant forward head position strains the muscles in your neck, leading to pain and stiffness. Stress also plays a significant role, causing your muscles to tense up and exacerbate the discomfort. Ergonomic issues, such as poorly designed workstations or improper sleeping positions, can further contribute to the problem.

Specific somatic exercises can be incredibly effective in addressing neck pain.

1. Neck Rolls

- **Instructions**: Sit or stand comfortably and slowly drop your chin toward your chest. Gently roll your head to the right, bringing your ear toward your shoulder. Circle your head back and to the left, then return to the starting position. Repeat five times in each direction.
- **Cue**: Keep the movement slow and controlled. Focus on the stretch and the sensations in your neck.

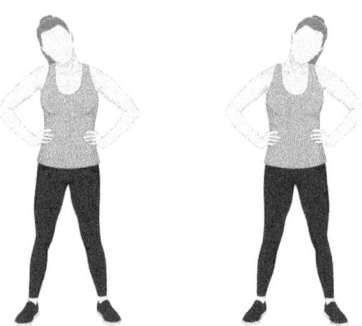

2. Chin Tucks

- **Instructions**: While sitting or standing, look straight ahead and gently pull your head back, tucking your chin as if trying to create a double chin. Hold for five seconds, then relax. Repeat this exercise ten times.
- **Cue**: Keep your shoulders relaxed and avoid tilting your head up or down. This is a subtle movement but very effective for improving posture.

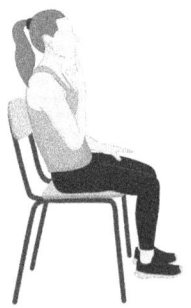

3. Upper Trapezius Stretch

- **Instructions**: Sit or stand with your back straight. Place your right hand on the left side of your head and gently pull your head toward your right shoulder. Hold for 20-30 seconds, then switch sides.
- **Cue**: Keep your shoulders down as you pull your head toward your shoulder. You should feel a gentle stretch along the side of your neck and upper shoulder.

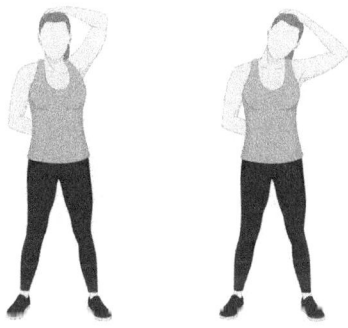

Each of these exercises targets different aspects of neck pain. Neck rolls improve neck mobility by gently stretching and relaxing the muscles. This can help release tension and increase your range of motion. Chin tucks strengthen the neck muscles, particularly those that support proper posture, helping to reduce the strain caused by forward head positions. The upper trapezius stretch focuses on releasing tension in the upper shoulders and the side of the neck, areas that commonly harbor stress-related tightness. Regularly practicing these exercises can alleviate pain and maintain better neck health.

Quick Tip:

Perform these exercises daily, especially if you spend long hours sitting at a desk or using electronic devices. Consistent practice will help alleviate pain and maintain better neck health over time.

A sample routine for neck pain relief might look like this:

1. **Neck rolls** - Begin with five in each direction, moving slowly and mindfully.
2. **Chin tucks** - Follow with ten, holding each position for five seconds.
3. **Upper trapezius stretch** - Finish with holding each side for 20-30 seconds.

To manage and prevent neck pain, aim to practice this routine daily, preferably in the morning or evening

If you spend a lot of time at a desk, consider integrating these exercises into short breaks throughout the day. This can help keep your neck muscles relaxed and reduce the buildup of tension, making your workday more comfortable and productive.

SOMATIC EXERCISES FOR HEADACHE RELIEF

Headaches can be an all-too-frequent companion, often sneaking up on you when you least expect it. Stress, muscle tension, and poor posture are some of the most common culprits. Tension headaches, in particular, result from tight muscles in your neck, shoulders, and scalp. They create a sensation of a tight band squeezing around your head. Stress and anxiety exacerbate this, causing your body to tense up further. This tension often radiates from the neck and shoulders, areas prone to stress-related tightness. Poor posture, especially from prolonged sitting or looking down at devices, can strain these muscles, making headaches more likely.

To alleviate headache pain, you can incorporate several effective somatic exercises into your routine.

1. Neck Rolls and Stretches

- **Instructions**: Sit comfortably, drop your chin toward your chest, and slowly roll your head to the right, bringing your ear toward your shoulder. Then, roll your head to the left. Repeat this five times in each direction. Then place your right hand on the left side of your head and gently pull your head toward your right shoulder. Hold for 20-30 seconds then switch sides.
- **Cue**: Keep the movement slow and smooth, feeling a gentle stretch along the sides of your neck.

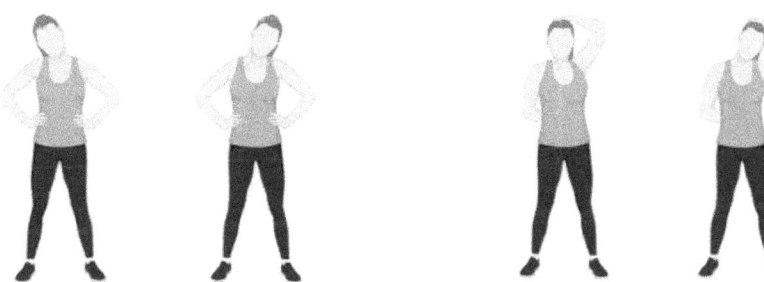

2. Shoulder Shrugs and Rolls

- **Instructions**: Stand or sit with your back straight. Shrug your shoulders up toward your ears, hold for a moment, then release them down. Afterward, perform forward and backward shoulder rolls. Shrug and roll your shoulders for 10-15 seconds in each direction.

- **Cue**: As you release your shoulders, exhale deeply to help release tension.

3. Scalp, Forehead, and Temple Massage

- **Instructions**: Using your fingertips, gently massage your scalp in circular motions. Slowly work your way down to your forehead and temples, massaging these areas to release tension. Spend 1-2 minutes on each area.
- **Cue**: Apply gentle pressure, focusing on any areas of tightness or discomfort. This technique helps to improve blood flow and relieve tightness.

4. Shoulder Blade Massage

- **Instructions**: Reach across your body with one hand to the opposite shoulder blade. Use your fingers to knead the muscles there, applying pressure to release deep-seated tension.
- **Cue**: Move slowly, applying as much pressure as feels comfortable to release tension in the muscles.

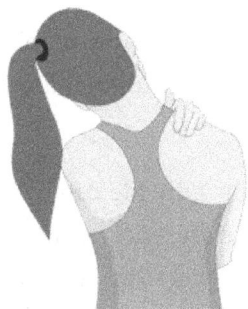 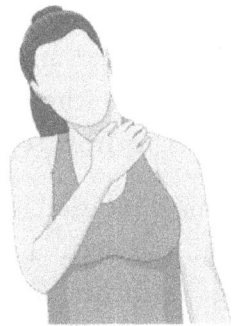

5. Breathing Exercises for Relaxation

- **Instructions**: Sit or lie down comfortably, close your eyes, and take slow, deep breaths. Focus on the rise and fall of your abdomen with each breath. You can try breathing techniques like **Box Breathing** (inhale for 4 seconds, hold for 4 seconds, exhale for 4 seconds, hold for 4 seconds), **4-7-8 Breathing** (inhale for 4, hold for 7, exhale for 8), or **Heart-Centered Breathing** (focusing on breathing deeply into your chest). Continue for 2-3 minutes.
- **Cue**: Concentrate on the breath, and let your body relax with each exhale.

Quick Tip:

Perform these techniques at the onset of a headache or incorporate them into your routine to prevent tension from building up. Breathing exercises can be done anytime, anywhere to help you manage stress throughout the day.

These exercises offer numerous benefits for headache relief and overall well-being. By reducing muscle tension, you alleviate one of the primary causes of tension headaches. Improved blood flow and circulation to your neck and head help reduce the frequency and intensity of headaches. Additionally, these movements promote enhanced relaxation and mental clarity, making it easier to manage stress and anxiety. The combination of physical and mental relaxation techniques can provide immediate relief and prevent headaches from recurring.

Incorporating these exercises into your daily life can be simple and effective and can make a significant difference in managing and preventing headaches. Perform the exercises at the onset of headache symptoms to provide immediate relief. Integrate these movements into your morning and evening routines to maintain muscle flexibility and reduce the likelihood of tension buildup. Using these exercises as a preventive measure during particularly stressful periods can also be beneficial. For instance, if you have a long day of work ahead, taking a few minutes to perform these exercises can help you stay relaxed and focused. By understanding the common causes of headaches and using targeted somatic exercises, you can find relief and improve your overall quality of life.

SOMATIC SOLUTIONS FOR SHOULDER PAIN

Shoulder pain is a common issue many people face, often due to our modern lifestyles. Statistics show that up to 67% of people will experience shoulder pain at some point in their lives. This pain can stem from various causes, including repetitive motions, injuries, and poor posture. For example, activities like typing on a computer, lifting heavy objects, or even sleeping in an awkward position can strain the shoulder muscles. Injuries such as rotator cuff tears or dislocations are common culprits. Additionally, stress can lead to muscle tension in the shoulders, exacerbating any existing discomfort.

Incorporating specific somatic exercises into your routine can be incredibly beneficial to manage shoulder pain effectively.

1. Shoulder Blade Squeeze

- **Instructions**: Sit or stand with your back straight. Gently squeeze your shoulder blades together as if trying to hold a pencil between them. Hold this position for five seconds, then release. Repeat this movement ten times.
- **Cue**: Keep your shoulders relaxed and avoid lifting them toward your ears. Focus on the movement between your shoulder blades.

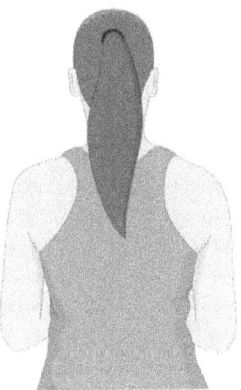
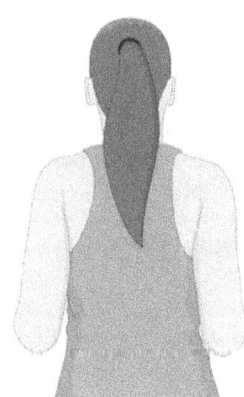

2. Arm Circles

- **Instructions**: Stand with your feet shoulder-width apart and extend your arms out to your sides at shoulder height. Make small circles with your arms, gradually increasing the size of the circles. Perform this exercise for 30 seconds in each direction.
- **Cue**: Keep your arms straight and controlled, and focus on smooth, continuous movements as you increase the size of the circles.

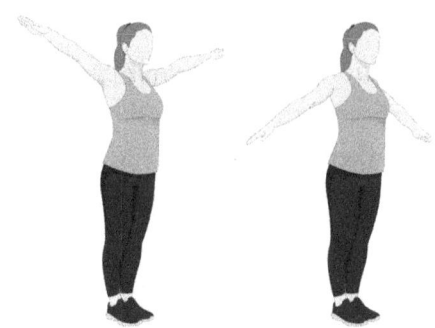

3. Cross-Body Shoulder Stretch

- **Instructions**: Bring one arm across your body and use your opposite hand to gently press the arm closer to your chest. Hold this stretch for 20-30 seconds, then switch sides.
- **Cue**: Keep your shoulder relaxed as you stretch, focusing on feeling the release of tension across your upper back and shoulder.

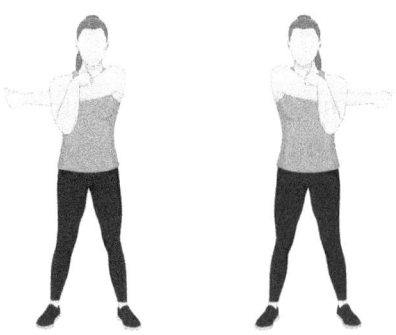

Quick Tip:

Perform these exercises daily, especially after long periods of sitting or working at a desk. Regular practice can help maintain shoulder mobility and prevent future discomfort.

Each of these exercises offers unique benefits for alleviating shoulder pain. Shoulder blade squeezes are particularly effective for strengthening the upper back muscles, which provide essential support for the shoulders. This exercise helps improve posture and reduces the strain on the shoulder joints. Arm circles enhance shoulder joint mobility by promoting a full range of motion. This increased mobility can help prevent stiffness and improve overall shoulder function. The cross-body shoulder stretch targets the muscles that often become tight and tense, providing a deep stretch that helps release built-up tension.

A sample routine for shoulder pain relief might look like this:

1. **Shoulder blade squeezes** - Start with ten focusing on the contraction and release of the muscles.
2. **Arm circles** - Follow with 30 seconds in each direction to improve joint mobility.
3. **Cross-body shoulder stretch** - Finish with holding each side for 20-30 seconds.

Aim to practice this routine daily, preferably in the morning or when you feel shoulder tension building up. You can also integrate these exercises into short breaks throughout your day, especially if you spend long hours at a desk. This routine can help maintain shoulder flexibility, reduce pain, and improve overall shoulder health.

MANAGING JOINT PAIN WITH SOMATIC EXERCISES

Joint pain can be a debilitating condition, affecting your ability to perform even the simplest tasks. Common causes of joint pain include arthritis, which involves inflammation of the joints, leading to stiffness and pain. Overuse injuries are another frequent cause, often resulting from repetitive activities that place undue stress on the joints. Inflammation, whether due to autoimmune conditions or acute injuries, can exacerbate the discomfort, making movement painful and challenging. Understanding these causes helps address the root of the problem and find effective solutions through somatic exercises.

Incorporating specific somatic exercises into your routine can be highly beneficial to manage joint pain effectively. Gentle range-of-motion exercises are an excellent starting point. These movements help maintain joint flexibility and prevent stiffness. For example, if you experience knee pain, try:

1. Seated Leg Extensions

- **Instructions**: Sit on a chair with your feet flat on the ground. Slowly extend one leg, straightening it as much as possible without causing pain. Hold for a few seconds, then return to the starting position. Repeat this movement 10-15 times on each leg.
- **Cue**: Keep your movements slow and controlled, focusing on maintaining good posture as you extend your leg.

PAIN MANAGEMENT | 85

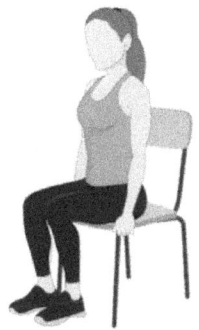 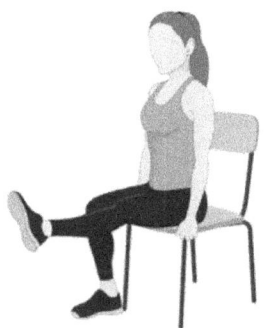

Isometric contractions are another valuable technique. These exercises involve contracting the muscles around the joint without actually moving the joint, which helps strengthen muscles without placing strain on the joints.

2. Isometric Shoulder Presses

- **Instructions**: Stand with your back against a wall, arms straight at your side. Press your palms into the wall, engaging the muscles around your shoulder. Hold this contraction for 10 seconds, then release. Repeat this exercise 5-10 times.
- **Cue**: Focus on activating the muscles without moving your shoulder. This will strengthen the muscles without placing stress on the joint.

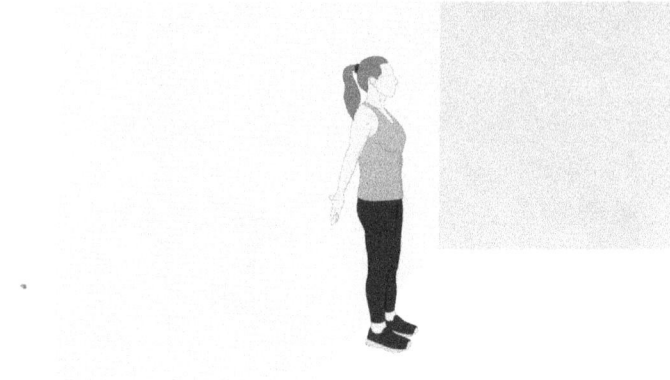

3. Low-Impact Aerobic Exercises

- **Description**: Exercises like swimming and cycling are great for joint health. They promote circulation, improve flexibility, and keep the joints moving without causing pain or strain.
- **Cue**: Aim for 20-30 minutes of low-impact aerobic activity, such as swimming or cycling, to enhance joint health and overall mobility.

Quick Tip:

Incorporate these exercises into your daily routine to improve joint health over time. Focus on gentle movements and controlled contractions to avoid any additional strain on your joints.

Each type of exercise offers distinct benefits for alleviating joint pain. Range-of-motion exercises are crucial for maintaining joint flexibility, reducing the risk of stiffness, and improving overall mobility. Isometric contractions help strengthen the muscles surrounding the joints, providing better support and reducing the likelihood of further injury. Low-impact aerobic exercises increase blood flow to the joints, which helps reduce inflammation and promote healing. These exercises also improve your overall cardiovascular health, contributing to a sense of well-being.

A sample routine for joint pain relief could look like this:

1. **Seated leg extensions** - Start with 10-15 to warm up and improve knee flexibility.
2. **Isometric shoulder presses** - Follow with 5-10 to strengthen the shoulder muscles.
3. **Low-impact aerobic exercise** -Incorporate 20-30 minutes such as cycling or swimming, to enhance overall joint health.

Aim to practice this routine at least three times a week, gradually increasing the duration and intensity as your comfort level improves. Remember to listen to your body and adjust the exercises as needed to avoid causing further pain. By consistently practicing these somatic exercises, you can manage joint pain effectively and improve your overall quality of life.

DEVELOPING A PERSONALIZED PAIN MANAGEMENT PLAN

Creating a personalized pain management plan is vital because each person's experience with pain is unique. What works for one person may not work for another. This individuality stems from differences in pain thresholds, underlying conditions, and even emotional responses to pain. Tailored strategies are necessary to address these variations effectively. A customized plan ensures that the exercises and techniques you use are specifically suited to your needs, making them more effective and easier to stick with over time. By focusing on your unique pain experience, you can develop a plan that brings genuine relief and improves your quality of life.

To develop a personalized pain management plan, start by assessing your specific pain areas. Take note of where you feel the most discomfort and consider any patterns you notice. For example, do you experience more pain in the morning or after certain activities? This self-assessment will help you identify the primary areas to target. Next, set realistic goals. These could include reducing pain levels, improving mobility, or increasing the duration of pain-free periods. Clear, achievable goals provide motivation and a sense of direction. Once your goals are set, choose appropriate exercises that align with them. For instance, if you experience lower back pain, focus on exercises that target that area, like pelvic tilts and Cat-Cow stretches.

Tracking your progress is crucial for maintaining and adjusting your plan. Don't forget, you can find printable resources, including detailed guides, trackers, and journals in the free workbook located in the Bonus Material section at the front of this book.

Keeping a pain journal is an effective way to monitor your symptoms and the impact of your exercises. Note the intensity and location of your pain before and after each session, as well as any changes in your overall well-being. Regular self-assessments can help you identify patterns and adjust your plan as needed. For example, if you notice that a particular exercise consistently aggravates your pain, you can modify or replace it. Adjusting your exercises based on your progress ensures that your plan remains effective and responsive to your needs.

Additional resources and support can enhance your pain management plan. There are numerous books and articles on somatic exercises and pain management that provide valuable insights and techniques. Online communities and support groups offer a platform to share experiences, ask questions, and receive encouragement from others who understand what you're going through. Consulting healthcare professionals, such as physical therapists or pain specialists, can provide personalized advice and additional strategies for managing your pain. These professionals can help you refine your plan and ensure that you're using the most effective techniques for your specific situation.

By creating a personalized pain management plan, you take control of your well-being. This approach acknowledges the unique nature of your pain and provides a framework for effective, tailored management. By assessing your specific pain areas, setting realistic goals, choosing appropriate exercises, and tracking your progress, you can develop a plan that brings meaningful relief. Seeking additional resources and support further enhances your plan, providing you with the knowledge and encouragement needed to manage your pain effectively.

MAKE A DIFFERENCE WITH YOUR REVIEW!

SHARE THE POWER OF KINDNESS

"The best way to find yourself is to lose yourself in the service of others."

— MAHATMA GANDHI

People who give without expecting anything in return often live more joyful, fulfilling lives. Let's join together to make a difference!

Would you help someone just like you—someone curious about **Somatic Exercises** but unsure where to begin?

My goal is to make **Somatic Exercises** simple for everyone. Whether it's to ease stress, relieve pain, or build emotional strength, I want this book to reach as many people as possible. But to do that, I need your help.

Most readers choose books based on reviews, and your words could inspire someone to begin their own journey with **Somatic Exercises**. By leaving a review, you could be the reason someone finally finds relief from stress and tension.

Your review could help:

- ...one more teacher find calm in a busy day.
- ...one more person manage their pain with simple, mindful movements.

- …one more friend take control of their stress and emotions.
- …one more family member build resilience for a healthier life.

Making a difference is simple and only takes a minute. Just scan the QR code to leave your review:

If helping others is something you believe in, you're my kind of person. Thank you, from the bottom of my heart, for supporting this mission and for being a part of this journey!

- **Jackie Brown**

5

ENHANCING EMOTIONAL RESILIENCE

There was a time when I felt completely overwhelmed by life's demands. Juggling work, family, and personal commitments left me feeling drained and emotionally fragile. One evening, after a particularly tough day, I decided to try a simple somatic exercise I had read about. I lay on my mat, closed my eyes, and began focusing on my breath, allowing my body to unwind. As I moved through the gentle stretches and mindful breathing, I felt a wave of calm wash over me. That night, I realized somatic exercises could be a lifeline for emotional resilience.

THE ROLE OF SOMATIC EXERCISES IN EMOTIONAL HEALTH

Somatic exercises play a crucial role in regulating the nervous system. When you're stressed, your body shifts into a fight-or-flight mode, which can lead to a cascade of physical and emotional symptoms. By engaging in mindful movement, you activate the parasympathetic nervous system, which helps counteract this stress response. This activation promotes relaxation, reduces anxiety, and creates a sense of inner calm. One of the key benefits of somatic exercises is their impact on cortisol levels. Cortisol, often referred to as the stress hormone, can wreak havoc on your body and mind when levels remain elevated. Gentle, mindful movements help lower cortisol levels, reducing the harmful effects of chronic stress.

Moreover, somatic exercises enhance mood through the release of endorphins. These "feel-good" hormones elevate your emotional state, making you feel happier and more energized. Unlike high-intensity workouts that sometimes leave you exhausted, somatic exercises provide a gentle way to boost your mood without straining your body. This combination of relaxation and endorphin release creates a powerful tool for improving emotional well-being.

Building emotional resilience is essential for managing life's inevitable ups and downs. Emotional resilience allows you to bounce back from adversity, handle stress more effectively, and maintain a positive outlook even in challenging times. Practicing somatic exercises regularly enhances your ability to regulate emotions, leading to improved mental clarity and focus. This heightened state of awareness helps you navigate stressful situations with greater ease. Additionally, emotional resilience contributes to greater overall life satisfaction. When you feel equipped to handle whatever comes your way, you experience a deeper sense of fulfillment and joy.

Scientific research supports the role of somatic exercises in promoting emotional health. Studies have shown that movement can significantly impact mood and emotional regulation. For instance, research on the effects of acute exercise indicates that even a single session of physical activity can enhance mood and cognitive functions. The release of neurochemicals like endorphins and the increased blood flow to the brain contribute to these positive effects. Additionally, somatic exercises have been found to positively influence stress hormones, further supporting their role in emotional regulation. Expert testimonials also highlight the transformative power of these practices. Practitioners often report significant improvements in their clients' emotional well-being after incorporating somatic exercises into their routines.

One of my friends, Amanda, struggled with severe anxiety that often left her feeling paralyzed. Traditional therapy and medication provided some relief, but she still felt overwhelmed by her emotions. I introduced her to somatic exercises, starting with simple breathwork and gentle stretches. Over time, Amanda noticed a significant reduction in her anxiety levels. The practice helped her connect with her body, providing a sense of control and calm that she hadn't experienced before. Another powerful example is my own journey. During a particularly difficult period of my life, I turned to somatic exercises as a way to cope with the emotional turmoil. The mindful movements and focused breathing helped me process my emotions, leading to a profound sense of emotional recovery.

Incorporating somatic exercises into your routine can have a transformative impact on your emotional health. By regulating the nervous system, reducing stress hormones, and enhancing mood, these practices provide a holistic approach to building emotional resilience. The benefits extend beyond immediate stress relief, offering long-term improvements in mental clarity, focus, and overall life satisfaction. Whether you're dealing with anxiety or stress or simply looking to enhance your emotional well-being, somatic exercises offer a gentle yet powerful solution.

TECHNIQUES FOR MANAGING EMOTIONAL STRESS

Mindfulness-based stress reduction is an incredible technique that integrates seamlessly with somatic exercises to manage emotional stress. I've found that combining mindful practices with physical movement can create a profound sense of calm and presence. Mindful breathing is one such practice. It involves focusing on your breath and noticing the sensations as you inhale and exhale. This simple act can anchor you in the present moment, reducing the mental chatter that often fuels stress. Body scan meditation is another powerful tool. By systematically bringing attention to different parts of your body, you can identify areas of tension and consciously release them. Grounding techniques, like feeling your feet on the floor or focusing on the sensation of your hands touching each other, can also be incredibly effective in bringing you back to the present moment when stress starts to build.

Specific somatic exercises for stress relief can make a significant difference in how you feel. Next we will talk about progressive muscle relaxation and stretching with mindful awareness.

Progressive Muscle Relaxation Technique

1. **Lie down** in a comfortable position, allowing your body to relax.
2. **Begin with your toes**:
    - Tense the muscles in your toes for a few seconds.
    - Slowly release the tension and relax.
3. **Move to your calves**:
    - Tense the muscles in your calves, hold for a few seconds.
    - Release the tension and let them relax.

1. **Progress to your thighs**:
   - Tense the muscles in your thighs, hold briefly.
   - Slowly release the tension.
2. **Continue moving up your body**, focusing on each muscle group:
   - Tense the muscles in each area for a few seconds, then release the tension.
3. **Cover your entire body**, including your abdomen, chest, arms, and face, allowing each muscle group to fully relax.

By the end of the exercise, your entire body should feel more relaxed and tension-free.

Gentle Stretching with Mindful Awareness

1. **Start by stretching your arms overhead**:
   - Reach up slowly, feeling the stretch through your arms, shoulders, and sides.
   - Hold this position for a few deep breaths, paying attention to how your body feels.
2. **Slowly bend forward**:
   - Gently hinge at your hips, allowing your arms to fall forward towards the ground.
   - Feel the stretch in your back, hamstrings, and legs.
3. **Hold each stretch for a few breaths**:
   - Focus on your breathing, inhaling deeply and exhaling slowly.
   - Allow your muscles to relax and lengthen with each breath.
4. **Move mindfully**:
   - Pay attention to the sensations in your body as you stretch, avoiding any discomfort.

- Let your breath guide you, helping you deepen the stretch without forcing it.

This practice promotes relaxation and flexibility, allowing you to connect with your body through mindful movement.

Consistency is crucial when it comes to managing stress effectively. Establishing a regular routine helps you make these practices a part of your daily life rather than something you only do when you feel overwhelmed. Set aside dedicated time each day for your somatic exercises. Whether it's first thing in the morning, during a lunch break, or before bed, find a time that works for you and stick to it. This consistency helps reinforce the habit, making it easier to turn to these techniques when you need them most. Over time, you'll find that consistent practice not only reduces your immediate stress levels but also builds your resilience to future stressors.

Integrating these exercises into your daily life can be simple. One practical way to incorporate mindfulness is during daily chores. When washing dishes, focus on the sensation of the warm water and the texture of the soap. Use these moments as opportunities for mindful practice. Brief breaks at work can also be an excellent time for stress-relief exercises. Take a few minutes to practice mindful breathing or do some gentle stretches at your desk. These short breaks can help reset your mind and body, making you more focused and productive. Integrating mindful movement into your morning routine can set a positive tone for the day. Spend a few minutes stretching and focusing on your breath before you start your day. This practice can help you feel grounded and ready to handle whatever comes your way.

EXERCISES TO BOOST MOOD AND POSITIVITY

Movement has an incredible ability to uplift your mood and infuse your day with positivity. When you move your body, you release endorphins, often referred to as "happy hormones." These natural chemicals interact with the receptors in your brain, reducing your perception of pain and triggering a positive feeling in the body. It's similar to the high you get after a good run or a satisfying workout. Movement also helps reduce stress hormones like cortisol, which can accumulate and cause feelings of anxiety or depression. By moving, you create a physiological shift that promotes relaxation and happiness.

One of the most empowering aspects of somatic exercises is how they can improve self-esteem through heightened body awareness. When you become more attuned to your body, you start to appreciate its capabilities and potential. This awareness fosters a sense of pride and accomplishment, boosting your overall self-esteem. Imagine starting your day with a series of dynamic stretches. As you reach and extend, you feel your muscles waking up and your blood flowing. These movements not only prepare your body for the day ahead but also set a positive tone, making you feel more confident and ready to tackle any challenges.

To elevate your mood, try incorporating specific mood-boosting exercises into your routine. Dynamic stretching routines are a great place to start.

1. Dynamic Arm and Leg Swings

- **Instructions**: Begin by standing with your feet shoulder-width apart. Gently swing your arms forward and backward, gradually increasing the range of motion. After

10-15 swings, move on to leg swings. Stand on one leg and gently swing the other leg forward and backward. Repeat on the opposite leg.
- **Cue**: Focus on controlled, rhythmic movements, allowing your body to warm up and your blood to circulate.

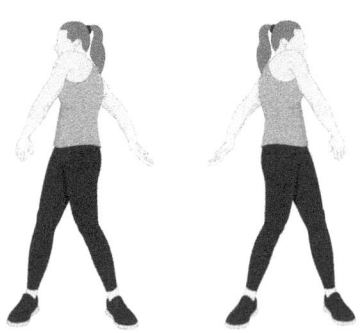

2. Somatic Dance or Free Movement

- **Instructions**: Put on your favorite music and allow your body to move freely. There's no right or wrong way to do this—just let your body express itself through movement. Dance for 2-5 minutes, focusing on how the music makes you feel.
- **Cue**: Move however feels natural and enjoyable, focusing on the joy of movement rather than form.

3. Joyful Jumping Exercises

- **Instructions**: Start with small jumps, focusing on the sensation of your feet leaving and returning to the ground. As you become more comfortable, incorporate arm movements, like reaching up towards the sky as you jump.

Continue jumping for 30-60 seconds, gradually increasing the height and intensity.
- **Cue**: Stay light on your feet and let your movements feel playful and fun. Imagine shaking off any negative energy as you jump.

4. Incorporating Gratitude

- **Instructions**: After completing your mood-boosting exercises, take a moment to reflect on what you're grateful for. You can either sit quietly and think about these things, or write them down in a gratitude journal. Focus on the positive feelings that gratitude brings. You can download the included gratitude journals by scanning the QR code located in the Bonus Section in the front of the book.
- **Cue**: Let the feeling of gratitude fill your body, enhancing the positive energy created through movement.

Quick Tip:

Incorporate these exercises into your daily routine to maintain a positive mindset and lift your spirits whenever you're feeling low. Adding music and gratitude can further amplify the benefits of these joyful movements.

Before or after your somatic exercises, take a few minutes to jot down three things you're grateful for. This practice shifts your focus from what's lacking to what's abundant in your life, fostering a sense of contentment and happiness. You can also integrate positive affirmations during movement. As you stretch or dance, repeat affirmations like "I am strong," "I am capable," or "I am grateful." These positive statements reinforce a healthy mindset, enhancing the emotional benefits of the exercises.

Real-life experiences highlight the profound impact of these practices. One of my students, Lisa, struggled with depression for years. Traditional therapies offered limited relief, so she decided to try somatic exercises. She started with dynamic stretching and free movement, gradually incorporating gratitude journaling. Over time, Lisa noticed significant improvements in her mood and outlook on life. She felt more energized, positive, and connected to her body. Another community member shared how joyful jumping exercises transformed their mornings, helping them start each day with a burst of happiness and enthusiasm. These stories underscore the transformative power of somatic exercises, offering a pathway to greater emotional well-being and positivity.

BUILDING MENTAL RESILIENCE THROUGH MOVEMENT

Mental resilience is your ability to recover from setbacks, adapt to change, and navigate challenges with a clear mind. It's a critical skill that allows you to bounce back from adversity and handle life's ups and downs more effectively. When you cultivate mental resilience, you enhance your problem-solving skills, making it easier to find solutions even in stressful situations. This adaptability is vital in today's fast-paced world, where change is constant and often unpredictable.

One effective way to build mental resilience is through balance and coordination exercises. These exercises challenge your body and mind, requiring you to focus and maintain stability. Simple practices include:

1. Standing on One Leg

- **Instructions**: Stand on one leg for 30 seconds, then switch to the other leg. Once you feel stable, try closing your eyes

to add an extra challenge. This exercise not only strengthens your balance but also trains your mind to remain focused and calm under pressure.
- **Cue**: Keep your core engaged and focus on a fixed point to help with balance. If closing your eyes, visualize staying steady.

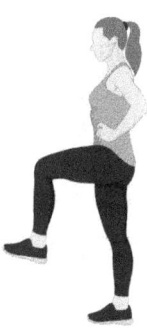

Challenging yet achievable physical tasks are a great way to build mental resilience. Set small, attainable goals that push you out of your comfort zone without overwhelming you.

2. Plank Position

- **Instructions**: Start in a plank position, keeping your body in a straight line from head to heels. Hold for 30 seconds longer than usual, gradually increasing your endurance. This exercise challenges both your mental resilience and physical strength, helping you push past discomfort and build confidence.
- **Cue**: Engage your core and focus on maintaining a strong, straight posture. Breathe deeply to stay calm and grounded as the challenge increases.

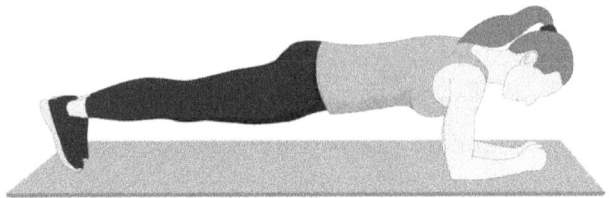

Quick Tip:

Set small, achievable goals for each exercise and gradually increase the difficulty over time. Each time you extend your limits, you're building both mental and physical resilience, proving to yourself that you can overcome obstacles with focus and determination.

These tasks help build confidence and resilience, proving to yourself that you can overcome challenges and achieve your goals.

Developing mental resilience through somatic exercises offers several key benefits. Better stress management is one of the most significant advantages. When you're more resilient, you're better equipped to handle stress without becoming overwhelmed. Increased emotional stability is another benefit. By regularly engaging in mindful movement, you train your mind to remain calm and composed, even in the face of adversity. This stability allows you to navigate emotional ups and downs with greater ease. Ultimately, greater overall well-being is the most rewarding benefit. When you're mentally resilient, you experience a deeper sense of satisfaction and fulfillment, knowing you can handle whatever life throws your way.

To help you build mental resilience, start with weekly goals and routines that gradually increase in complexity. Begin with basic balance exercises and mindful movement practices, then incorporate more challenging tasks as you progress. Track your progress by keeping a journal of your experiences. Note any improvements in your balance, coordination, and emotional stability. This record will serve as a source of motivation and encouragement, showing you how far you've come. Staying motivated can be challenging, but setting small, achievable goals can help. Celebrate your successes, no matter how small, and remind yourself of the benefits you're gaining. Surround yourself with supportive individuals who encourage your efforts and share in your journey towards greater mental resilience.

SOMATIC PRACTICES FOR EMOTIONAL RELEASE

Emotional release is a profound process where stored emotions are expressed and released through movement. Our bodies often hold onto emotions, creating physical tension that can manifest as tight muscles, aches, or even chronic pain. This connection between physical and emotional tension is why somatic exercises are so effective. You can tap into these stored emotions and release them by engaging in specific movements, leading to significant emotional relief and well-being.

1. Somatic Shaking

- **Instructions**: Stand with your feet hip-width apart and your knees slightly bent. Begin by gently shaking your hands and arms, allowing the movement to spread throughout your body. Let your head move freely and feel the vibrations flow through your muscles. Continue for 1-2 minutes, focusing on how the movement releases tension and emotions.
- **Cue**: Don't worry about how you look—focus on the sensations and the sense of freedom as you shake. Feel the vibrations traveling through your body, helping to release stored energy and emotions.

2. Breathwork and Gentle Stretches

- **Instructions**: Pair deep, diaphragmatic breathing with gentle stretches. As you inhale deeply, raise your arms overhead. As you exhale, bend forward and let your arms and head hang loosely. Continue this movement for 1-2 minutes, using your breath to guide each stretch. This practice helps open up your body, allowing emotions to surface and be released.
- **Cue**: Focus on the rhythm of your breath, allowing each inhale to expand your body and each exhale to release any tension or emotions.

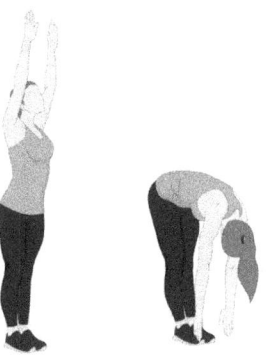

3. Vocalization for Emotional Release

- **Instructions**: As you move through stretches or shaking exercises, allow yourself to vocalize. This could be a deep sigh, a hum, or even a louder vocalization like a yell or a moan. The sound vibrations resonate through your body, helping to release deep-seated emotions. Try pairing a sigh with an exhale, or hum as you stretch. Practice this for 1-2

minutes, letting your voice flow naturally with your movements.
- **Cue**: Don't hold back—let your voice guide the release of emotions. Feel the resonance of your voice travel through your body, amplifying the emotional release.

Quick Tip:

Practice these exercises regularly to help release emotional tension as it builds. Create a safe, comfortable space where you can fully engage with the movements and allow your emotions to flow freely.

The benefits of emotional release through somatic exercises are profound. Releasing stored emotions can lead to a significant reduction in emotional tension. You may find that you feel more relaxed and at ease, both physically and emotionally. Greater emotional clarity is another benefit. By releasing emotions, you make space for clearer thinking and better emotional regulation. You'll find it easier to understand and process your feelings, leading to healthier emotional responses. An enhanced sense of freedom often accompanies emotional release. When you let go of stored emotions, you free yourself from their hold, allowing for a more open and authentic experience of life.

Consider the story of David, who had been carrying the weight of unresolved grief for years. Traditional therapies hadn't fully addressed his needs, so he turned to somatic practices. Through regular sessions of somatic shaking and breathwork, David began to release the deep-seated grief that had been affecting his well-being. He described the experience as a breakthrough, feeling a sense of lightness and clarity he hadn't felt in years.

Another relatable story was Maria's finding that vocalization during her somatic exercises helped her release anger and frustration. The act of vocalizing her emotions allowed her to process them in a safe and controlled way, leading to significant emotional relief.

These stories highlight the transformative power of emotional release through somatic exercises. By engaging in practices like somatic shaking, breathwork combined with movement, and vocalization, you can tap into stored emotions and release them, leading to improved emotional health. The reduction in emotional tension, greater emotional clarity, and enhanced sense of freedom are just a few of the benefits you can expect. Whether you're dealing with grief, anger, or any other stored emotions, somatic exercises offer a gentle yet powerful way to find relief and healing.

CREATING AN EMOTIONAL RESILIENCE ROUTINE

Having a consistent emotional resilience routine is like building muscle; the more you practice, the stronger you become. Creating this routine helps you develop habits that support sustained emotional health. When you know what to expect each day, it reduces uncertainty and provides a sense of stability. This predictability is comforting and can significantly alleviate anxiety. The psychological benefits of a routine cannot be overstated. It creates a structured environment where you can focus on your well-being without distractions, fostering a sense of control and empowerment.

To create an effective emotional resilience routine, start by choosing exercises that resonate with you. This could include somatic practices like gentle stretching, breathwork, or even a simple walk in nature. The key is to select activities that you enjoy and find relaxing. Setting a regular practice time is also crucial. Consistency is key, whether it's first thing in the morning, during a midday break, or before bed. When you practice at the same time each day, it becomes a natural part of your routine. Incorporating mindfulness and relaxation techniques can further enhance your routine. Practices like meditation, mindful breathing, or even listening to calming music can deepen your sense of peace and emotional balance.

You might find that different times of day call for different types of routines. For a morning routine aimed at emotional resilience, consider starting with a few minutes of mindful breathing to center yourself. Follow this with gentle stretches to wake up your body and perhaps a brief gratitude practice to set a positive tone for the day. This combination of activities helps ground you, making it easier to face the day's challenges with a calm and focused mind. On the other hand, an evening routine for emotional release might involve somatic exercises designed to release the day's accumulated tension. Start with a body scan meditation to identify areas of tightness, then move through a series of gentle stretches, focusing on your breath. Finish with a calming activity, like journaling or reading, to wind down and prepare for restful sleep.

Maintaining consistency is often the most significant challenge when establishing a new routine. Setting reminders can be incredibly helpful. Use your phone or a calendar app to schedule your practice times and set alerts to keep you on track. Tracking your progress with a journal can also provide motivation. Note how you feel before and after each session, any changes in your emotional state, and any insights you gain. This record serves as a tangible reminder of the benefits you're experiencing, reinforcing your commitment to the routine. You can download a free tracker journal located in the Bonus Section in the front of the book. Finding a practice buddy can add an extra layer of accountability.

Whether it's a friend, family member, or someone you connect with online, sharing your progress and supporting each other can make a significant difference.

Consistency in your emotional resilience routine builds the foundation for lasting emotional health. By choosing appropriate exercises, setting a regular practice time, and incorporating mindfulness and relaxation techniques, you create a routine that supports your well-being. Sample routines tailored to different times of day provide flexibility, allowing you to adapt your practice to your needs. Strategies like setting reminders, tracking progress, and finding a practice buddy help maintain consistency, ensuring that your routine becomes a natural and rewarding part of your daily life.

WEEKLY ROUTINES FOR EMOTIONAL RESILIENCE

Creating and following weekly routines for emotional resilience can provide lasting results. Consistent practice not only helps build emotional strength but also ensures that the benefits are long-term. By focusing on different emotional aspects each week, you can address various facets of emotional well-being comprehensively. Combining various somatic techniques within these routines ensures a holistic approach, making your practice more effective and engaging.

Week 1: Emotional Regulation & Mindfulness

Focus: Emotional regulation and mindfulness to build awareness and calmness.

- **Start with Mindful Breathing**: Spend a few minutes breathing deeply, focusing on the present moment.

- **Emotional Regulation Techniques**: Sit quietly, ask yourself how you're feeling, and acknowledge those emotions without judgment.
- **Gentle Stretches for Tension Release**: Focus on areas where you hold emotional stress (shoulders, neck).

Goal: By the end of the week, you should feel more in tune with your emotions and better equipped to manage them.

Week 2: Breathwork & Heart-Centered Breathing

Focus: Calming the nervous system and fostering emotional connection through breath.

- **Alternate Nostril Breathing**: Inhale through one nostril, close it, and exhale through the other. Repeat several cycles.
- **Heart-Centered Breathing**: Place your hand on your heart and imagine your breath flowing in and out of your chest.
- **Light Stretching**: Incorporate gentle stretches to integrate the benefits of breathwork into your body.

Goal: Cultivate a sense of compassion and connection with yourself through breath awareness.

Week 3: Body Scan Meditation & Grounding

Focus: Grounding and tuning into your body's sensations to release tension.

- **Body Scan Meditation**: Lie down comfortably and bring awareness to each part of your body, starting at your toes and moving to your head.

- **Grounding Exercise**: Stand with feet firmly planted and focus on the sensation of the earth beneath you.

Goal: Enhance your connection to the present moment and feel more centered and grounded.

Week 4: Emotional Release Through Movement

Focus: Releasing stored emotions with movement and vocalization.

- **Hip Openers**: Sit cross-legged and press your knees towards the floor, holding for a few breaths.
- **Pandiculation**: Stretch and contract your muscles slowly. For example, stretch your arms overhead, then curl into a fetal position.
- **Vocalization** (Optional): Allow natural sounds to emerge as you move, such as sighs or hums.

Goal: Release deep-seated emotions and tension stored in your body.

Quick Tips for Success:

- **Consistency is key—practice regularly for lasting benefits.**
- **Create a calm, comfortable space where you can fully engage in the exercises.**
- **Reflect on how each practice impacts your emotional and physical state.**

The benefits of following these weekly routines are profound. Consistent practice enhances emotional awareness and regulation, making it easier to manage stress and anxiety. By focusing on different emotional aspects each week, you develop a well-rounded approach to emotional health. The variety of somatic techniques keeps the practice engaging and ensures that you address multiple facets of emotional well-being. Over time, you'll find that these routines not only improve your emotional resilience but also contribute to greater overall well-being.

6

INTERACTIVE AND HOLISTIC APPROACHES

One evening, I sat at my desk, feeling utterly consumed by the endless responsibilities of work, family, and personal commitments. The pressure seemed unbearable, as if I was juggling too much, and I wondered how I could keep it all together and keep track of everything. That's when I decided to start tracking my progress. I grabbed a simple notebook and began jotting down my daily activities, exercises, and how I felt afterward. Over time, this practice became a lifeline, helping me stay motivated and accountable. Seeing my progress visualized on paper was incredible, and it gave me the push I needed to keep going.

TRACKING YOUR PROGRESS: JOURNALS AND TEMPLATES

Tracking your progress is a powerful tool to enhance motivation and accountability. Monitoring your practice allows you to visualize improvements over time, identify patterns and trends, and celebrate milestones and achievements. This process is not just about keeping records; it's about understanding your journey and recognizing your growth. Seeing your progress laid out before you can be incredibly motivating. It provides tangible evidence of your hard work and dedication, reinforcing the positive changes you're making in your life. This sense of achievement releases dopamine in your brain, a chemical that boosts your mood and encourages you to keep going.

There are various methods and tools you can use to track your progress. One of the simplest and most effective is a progress journal. This can be a blank notebook where you jot down your daily exercises, how you felt during and after the practice, and any observations or insights. You can also use tracking sheets and templates to systematically organize your entries. These templates can include sections for daily logs, weekly summaries, and monthly reflections.

To help you get started, let's look at some examples of tracking templates, which are included in the Bonus Section in the beginning of the book.

A daily practice log can include sections for the date, the exercises you performed, the duration of each exercise, and a space for notes or reflections. This log helps you keep track of your daily activities and notice any immediate changes or patterns.

A weekly progress summary can be used to reflect on your achievements over the past week. This template might include sections for what went well, challenges you faced, and goals for the upcoming week. This weekly reflection helps you see your progress in a broader context and make necessary adjustments to your practice.

A monthly reflection and goal-setting sheet can help you take a step back and look at the bigger picture. This template can include sections for summarizing your progress over the past month, setting new goals, and identifying any long-term trends or patterns.

Regular tracking offers numerous benefits. One of the most immediate is increased motivation and engagement. When you see your progress documented, it reinforces your commitment to your practice. You'll be more motivated to continue and less likely to skip sessions. Tracking your progress also provides a better understanding of your personal growth. By consistently monitoring your activities, you can identify what works best for you and what needs adjustment. This self-awareness helps you tailor your practice to your unique needs and goals.

Moreover, tracking enhances your ability to set and achieve goals. Regularly reviewing your progress and setting new objectives create a continuous cycle of improvement. This proactive approach keeps you focused and ensures that you're always moving forward.

REFLECTION SECTION: TRACKING YOUR PROGRESS

Take a moment to reflect on your current practice. Do you already track your progress? If not, how might starting this habit benefit you? Consider using the daily practice log templates provided in the **Bonus Section** to begin your tracking journey. Note how you feel before and after each session, the exercises you performed, and any observations or insights. Revisit this log at the end of the week to summarize your progress and set new goals. This simple practice can transform your approach to somatic exercises, making it more intentional and rewarding.

- Date:
- Exercises Performed:

- Duration:
- How I Felt Before:
- How I Felt After:
- Observations/Insights:

Tracking your progress is not just about keeping records; it's about understanding your journey and recognizing your growth. Visualizing improvements, identifying patterns, and celebrating milestones enhance your motivation and accountability, making your practice more effective and rewarding.

WORKSHEETS FOR SELF-REFLECTION

Self-reflection plays a crucial role in personal growth and progress within somatic exercises. It enhances self-awareness by allowing you to understand your body's responses, recognize areas of tension, and notice changes over time. This process provides valuable insights into your personal patterns and habits, helping you identify what works best for you and what might need adjustment. Moreover, self-reflection encourages mindful practice, ensuring that each session is intentional and focused. By regularly reflecting on your experiences, you can make informed decisions about your practice, leading to more effective and meaningful outcomes.

There are various types of interactive worksheets that can aid in this self-reflection process. One of the most beneficial tools is a daily reflection journal. This journal can include prompts such as "How did I feel before and after today's practice?" or "What specific areas of my body felt tense or relaxed?" These prompts guide you to think deeply about your experiences and document your observations. Another useful worksheet is a weekly progress assessment. This assessment can help you review your achievements over the past week, identify challenges, and set goals for the upcoming week. It encourages you to look at your practice from a broader perspective, helping you see the bigger picture. Emotion tracking charts are also valuable. These charts can help you monitor your emotional state throughout your practice, allowing you to see how somatic exercises impact your overall mood and well-being.

To effectively utilize these worksheets, set aside dedicated reflection time. This could be a few minutes at the end of each practice session or a longer period at the end of the week. Find a quiet space where you can focus without distractions. Be honest and thorough in your responses. The more detailed and sincere you are, the more valuable your reflections will be. Use your reflections to inform practice adjustments. If you notice that specific exercises consistently lead to tension or discomfort, consider modifying them or replacing them with alternatives. On the other hand, if you find certain movements particularly beneficial, make them a regular part of your routine.

Here are some sample worksheets that you can use to get started.

Daily Reflection Journal (Located in the Bonus Section)

- Date:
- How did I feel before today's practice?
- What exercises did I perform?
- How did I feel after today's practice?
- What specific areas of my body felt tense or relaxed?
- Any observations or insights?

Weekly Progress Assessment (Located in the Bonus Section)

- What went well this week?
- What challenges did I face?

- What did I learn about my body and practice?
- Goals for the upcoming week:

Emotion Tracking Chart (Located in the Bonus Section)

- Date:
- Emotion before practice: (e.g., anxious, calm, stressed)
- Emotion after practice:
- Notes on emotional changes:

Regular tracking and reflection offer numerous benefits. They increase motivation and engagement by providing tangible evidence of your progress. When you see your accomplishments documented, it reinforces your commitment to your practice. Reflection also enhances your understanding of personal growth. By consistently monitoring your experiences, you can identify patterns and trends, helping you make informed decisions about your practice. Additionally, regular reflection improves your ability to set and achieve goals. Regularly reviewing your progress and setting new objectives create a cycle of continuous improvement. This proactive approach keeps you focused and ensures that you're always moving forward.

INTEGRATING NUTRITION WITH SOMATIC PRACTICES

Proper nutrition is more than just fueling your body; it's about providing the right kind of energy that supports physical activity, muscle recovery, and mental clarity. When you eat well, your body has the energy it needs to perform exercises effectively. Nutrients like proteins support muscle recovery and growth, while vitamins and minerals ensure that your body functions optimally. This holistic approach enhances your physical performance and keeps your mind sharp and focused.

Balanced meals are the cornerstone of a healthy diet. Incorporate a variety of foods to ensure you're getting all the nutrients you need. Proteins, carbohydrates, and fats each play vital roles in your body. Proteins build and repair tissues, carbohydrates provide energy, and fats support cell function. Aim to fill half your plate with fruits and vegetables, a quarter with whole grains, and the remaining quarter with a source of lean protein. Hydration is equally important. Drinking enough water helps maintain fluid balance, supports digestion, and keeps your muscles hydrated. Try to drink at least eight glasses of water a day and more if you're engaging in intense physical activity. Timing your meals around your exercise routine can also make a big difference. Eating a light snack before exercising can provide the energy you need, while a balanced meal afterward helps with recovery.

Certain foods can offer additional benefits for your somatic health. Anti-inflammatory foods like turmeric and ginger can help reduce muscle soreness and inflammation, making recovery smoother. Foods rich in Omega-3 fatty acids, such as salmon and flaxseeds, support brain health and reduce inflammation, enhancing both physical and mental well-being. Hydrating fruits and vegetables like cucumber and watermelon not only keeps you hydrated but also provides essential vitamins and minerals. These foods nourish your body and mind, helping you get the most out of your somatic exercises.

To give you a clearer idea, let's look at some sample meal plans that align with your exercise routines.

Pre-exercise snack: consider a banana with a tablespoon of almond butter. This combination provides quick energy from the banana and sustained energy from the healthy fats in the almond butter.

Post-Workout: After your workout, a recovery meal might include grilled chicken, quinoa, and a side of steamed broccoli. The protein in the chicken helps repair muscles, while the quinoa provides complex carbohydrates for energy, and the broccoli offers essential vitamins and minerals.

Example Balanced daily meal plan:

- **Breakfast:** Greek yogurt topped with fresh berries and a drizzle of honey
- **Lunch:** quinoa salad with mixed greens, cherry tomatoes, cucumbers, and a lemon-tahini dressing.
- **Dinner:** A serving of baked salmon with a side of roasted sweet potatoes and sautéed spinach.

Integrating proper nutrition with your somatic practices not only enhances your physical performance but also supports your overall well-being. By paying attention to what you eat, staying hydrated, and timing your meals around your exercise routines, you provide your body with the fuel it needs to thrive. Including specific foods that support somatic health can further enhance the benefits, making your practice more effective and enjoyable. This holistic approach ensures that you're caring for both your body and mind, helping you achieve a balanced and healthy lifestyle.

IMPORTANCE OF SLEEP IN HOLISTIC HEALTH

I can still remember the nights I spent tossing and turning, unable to escape the clutches of insomnia. It wasn't until I made sleep a priority that I began to notice profound changes in my overall health. Sleep is a cornerstone of physical, mental, and emotional well-being. It supports muscle recovery, allowing your body to repair and grow stronger after the wear and tear of daily activities.

Without sufficient sleep, your muscles don't get the time they need to heal, leading to increased soreness and a higher risk of injury. A good night's sleep enhances cognitive function, sharpening your focus and improving memory. When you're well-rested, you can think more clearly, make better decisions, and be more productive. Sleep also plays a crucial role in regulating mood and stress levels. Lack of sleep can make you irritable and anxious, while adequate sleep helps you manage stress more effectively and maintain a balanced emotional state.

The connection between sleep and somatic practices is profound. Adequate sleep provides the energy needed for practice, making your sessions more effective and enjoyable. When you're well-rested, you have the stamina to engage fully in your exercises, allowing you to get the most out of each session. Improved focus and body awareness are other benefits of getting enough sleep. When your mind is clear, and your body is rested, you're more attuned to your movements and sensations, enhancing the effectiveness of your somatic exercises. Moreover, sleep enhances recovery and muscle repair, ensuring that your body is ready for the next practice session. By prioritizing sleep, you create a foundation that supports your somatic practice and overall health.

Improving sleep quality can be a transformative step toward better health. Establishing a regular sleep schedule is one of the most effective ways to improve sleep quality. Try to go to bed and wake up at the same time every day, even on weekends. This consistency helps regulate your body's internal clock, making it easier to fall asleep and wake up naturally. Creating a calming bedtime routine can also make a big difference. Engage in relaxing activities such as reading, taking a warm bath, or practicing gentle stretches before bed. These activities signal your body that it's time to wind down and prepare for sleep. Reducing screen time before bed is another important tip. The blue light emitted by phones, tablets, and computers can interfere with your body's production of melatonin, a hormone that regulates sleep. Try to avoid screens at least an hour before bedtime to help your body transition into sleep mode.

Incorporating a bedtime somatic exercise routine can further enhance your sleep quality. Start with gentle stretching exercises to release any tension that has built up over the day. Simple stretches like a forward bend or a gentle spinal twist can help relax your muscles and prepare your body for rest. Follow these stretches with relaxation techniques such as progressive muscle relaxation, where you tense and then release each muscle group, starting from your toes and working your way up to your head. This technique helps release physical tension and promotes a sense of calm. Finish your routine with breathwork to promote sleep. The 4-7-8 breathing technique is particularly effective. Inhale through your nose for a count of four, hold for a count of seven, and exhale through your mouth for a count of eight. Repeat this cycle a few times, focusing on the rhythm of your breath and allowing your mind to settle.

Taking these steps to improve your sleep quality can profoundly impact your overall health. By prioritizing sleep, you create a solid foundation that supports your physical, mental, and emotional well-being. This, in turn, enhances the effectiveness of your somatic exercises, allowing you to experience the full benefits of your practice.

USING SOMATIC TECHNIQUES IN EVERYDAY SITUATIONS

Somatic techniques are incredibly versatile, offering benefits that extend well beyond dedicated practice sessions. You can adapt these exercises to various daily situations, enhancing your overall quality of life and providing tools for immediate stress relief. Imagine waiting in a long line at the grocery store. Instead of becoming frustrated, you can engage in gentle weight shifting. Shift your weight from one foot to the other, paying close attention to how your body feels. This simple movement keeps you grounded and helps release tension, turning an otherwise tedious moment into an opportunity for mindfulness and relaxation.

Commuting can be another perfect time to incorporate somatic techniques. Whether you're on a bus, train, or carpool, seated breathing exercises can transform your commute into a calming experience. Focus on taking slow, deep breaths, filling your lungs completely and then exhaling fully. This practice helps reduce stress and prepares you for the day ahead or unwinds you after a long day. In addition, mindful movements and stretches can be seamlessly integrated into routine activities like cooking. While stirring a pot or chopping vegetables, take a moment to notice your posture. Are you standing straight? Are your shoulders relaxed? Incorporating gentle stretches, like rolling your shoulders or stretching your neck, can help you stay mindful and reduce physical tension.

Integrating somatic techniques into your daily life has numerous benefits. First and foremost, they help reduce everyday stress. By turning mundane moments into opportunities for mindfulness and movement, you diffuse the built-up tension that often accumulates throughout the day. Enhancing mindfulness and presence is another significant advantage. When you practice somatic techniques in everyday situations, you become more attuned to your body and surroundings. This heightened awareness fosters a deeper sense of presence, allowing you to fully experience and enjoy each moment.

Incorporating somatic techniques into your daily routine doesn't have to be complicated. Start by being mindful of your body posture and alignment throughout the day. Whether you're sitting at a desk, standing in line, or walking, pay attention to how you hold your body. Minor adjustments, like straightening your back or relaxing your shoulders, can make a big difference. Using triggers or reminders can also help you integrate these techniques naturally. Set phone notifications to remind you to take a deep breath or stretch every hour. These gentle nudges encourage you to pause and check in with your body, making somatic practices a regular part of your day.

Engaging in regular somatic practices in everyday situations enhances your overall well-being and makes these techniques second nature. Over time, you'll find that you naturally incorporate mindful movements and stretches without even thinking about it. This seamless integration helps you maintain a state of relaxation and mindfulness, even amidst the hustle and bustle of daily life. By being proactive and intentional, you can transform ordinary moments into opportunities for self-care and awareness, enriching your life in subtle yet profound ways.

As you continue to explore the versatility of somatic techniques, remember that the goal is to enhance your quality of life. These practices are not just exercises; they are tools for living more mindfully and joyfully. By incorporating somatic techniques into everyday situations, you create a foundation of well-being that supports you in all aspects of your life. Embrace these opportunities, and let them guide you toward a more balanced and fulfilling existence.

7

ADVANCED SUPPORT AND RESOURCES

One rainy afternoon, feeling overwhelmed and unable to focus, I tried something new: a guided audio meditation. I sat in my favorite chair, put on my headphones, and pressed play. The soothing voice guided me through a body scan, and for the first time in days, I felt a wave of calm wash over me. This experience opened my eyes to the power of audio guides, not just for meditation but for enhancing all aspects of my somatic practice.

UTILIZING AUDIO GUIDES FOR MEDITATION

Audio guides offer a unique advantage for meditation and somatic practices. They provide a structured, immersive experience that can significantly enhance your practice. Guided meditation is particularly beneficial for relaxation. Listening to a calm voice directing your focus helps you stay present and deeply engaged, reducing distractions and promoting a state of tranquility. Audio cues for body awareness are another powerful feature. They prompt you to notice specific sensations and areas of tension you might otherwise overlook. This heightened awareness can lead to more effective tension release and a deeper connection with your body. Additionally, the convenience of audio guides makes them perfect for on-the-go practice. Whether commuting, taking a walk, or simply sitting in a park, you can easily integrate a few minutes of mindful listening into your day.

There are various types of audio guides available, each catering to different aspects of meditation and somatic practice. Guided body scan meditations are excellent for systematically focusing on different parts of your body, helping you identify and release tension. Breathing exercises with audio prompts guide you through different breathing techniques, ensuring you maintain a steady rhythm and focus. Mindfulness and relaxation tracks are designed to help you unwind and center yourself, often featuring soothing music or nature sounds to enhance the experience. These different types of guides provide flexibility, allowing you to choose the one that best suits your needs at any given moment.

Accessing audio content is straightforward and convenient. Many websites and apps offer downloadable audio files specifically designed for meditation and somatic practices. Platforms like Insight Timer, Calm, and Headspace have extensive libraries of guided meditations and exercises. You can stream or download these files to your device, making them readily available whenever you need them. Creating an audio playlist can also be a great way to organize your favorite tracks. Compile a selection of body scans, breathing exercises, and relaxation tracks into a playlist that you can easily access, ensuring you have various options at your fingertips.

Using audio guides effectively requires a few simple strategies. First, using headphones can create an immersive experience, blocking out external distractions and allowing you to fully engage with the guided session. Setting aside dedicated time for audio-guided practice is also crucial. Whether it's a few minutes in the morning, during a lunch break, or before bed, having a consistent time slot can help establish a routine. Combining audio guides with physical exercises can offer a holistic approach to your practice. For example, you might start with a guided body scan followed by a series of gentle stretches, seamlessly integrating mindfulness with movement. This combination can enhance the benefits of both practices, leading to a more comprehensive and fulfilling experience.

CREATING YOUR OWN AUDIO PLAYLIST

Creating a personalized audio playlist can significantly enhance your practice. Start by exploring different types of audio content to find what resonates with you. Platforms like Insight Timer and Calm offer many options, from short breathing exercises to longer body scans. Once you've identified your favorites, compile them into a playlist that suits your needs. For instance, you might include:

- A 5-minute breathing exercise for quick stress relief.
- A 10-minute body scan for deeper relaxation.
- A 15-minute mindfulness track for a more extended practice session.

Organize your playlist in a way that flows naturally, starting with shorter exercises and gradually moving to longer sessions. This structure can help ease into your practice and build up to more intensive sessions. Having a well-curated playlist ensures you always have the right tool at your disposal, whether you need a quick reset or a deeper dive into relaxation.

Incorporating audio guides into your daily routine can transform your approach to somatic exercises and meditation. Their structured guidance, immersive experience, and convenience make them invaluable resources. Whether you're a beginner or looking to deepen your practice, audio guides can provide the support and direction you need to enhance your well-being.

REAL-LIFE SUCCESS STORIES AND TESTIMONIALS

When I first started exploring somatic exercises, I was skeptical. It's easy to doubt the effectiveness of something that seems so simple. However, hearing real-life success stories can make all the difference. These testimonials aren't just anecdotal; they are powerful reminders that transformation is possible. Seeing others' journeys—people who have faced similar struggles and found relief—can be incredibly inspiring and motivating. Relatable experiences provide proof that these exercises work, fostering an emotional connection and offering encouragement. Knowing that someone else has walked the same path and emerged stronger can give you the push you need to keep going.

Take Brian for instance. He was an avid runner who had to stop due to debilitating sciatic pain. After trying countless treatments with little success, he discovered clinical somatics. Within weeks, Brian experienced significant pain relief, allowing him to resume running and strength training. His story is a testament to the potential of somatic exercises to change lives. Similarly, Eve noted remarkable progress in both her body and mind just three weeks into her somatic practice. She felt more relaxed, her posture improved, and her chronic pain diminished. These stories underscore the effectiveness of somatic exercises in managing chronic pain and improving overall quality of life.

Stress and anxiety are common issues that many people face. Melanie found somatic exercises invaluable for de-stressing her body and relieving pain. She described how incorporating these practices helped her manage daily stressors more effectively, leading to a calmer, more balanced life. Another testimonial comes from Dan, an older skateboarder who suffered from chronic pain. Dan found significant relief and improved control over his body through somatic exercises. These accounts highlight the versatility of somatic practices in addressing both physical and emotional challenges.

Emotional resilience is another area where somatic exercises can make a significant impact. Libby, who had endured chronic pain for 15 years, found somatics transformative. Not only did her pain decrease, but she also felt healthier and happier, with a newfound emotional stability. Rhian, another practitioner, experienced incredible improvements in flexibility and pain relief, which positively affected her family life. These stories illustrate how somatic exercises can foster personal growth and transformation, helping individuals build emotional resilience and improve their relationships with others.

Hearing from beginners and advanced practitioners alike can be particularly motivating. For instance, Kathie avoided multi-level fusion surgery and regained her ability to hike and perform daily activities through somatic exercises. On the other end of the spectrum, Chris, who had been suffering from chronic pain for 19 years, found relief through consistent practice. These diverse experiences show that somatic exercises can benefit anyone, regardless of their starting point. Whether you are new to these practices or looking to deepen your existing routine, there is always room for growth and improvement.

The key takeaways from these stories are varied but unified by common themes. Techniques that worked well for individuals often involved:

- Consistent practice
- Mindful attention to the body's signals
- A willingness to adapt exercises to their specific needs

Overcoming common challenges, such as initial skepticism or difficulty maintaining a routine, required persistence and an open mind. Personal growth and transformation were frequently mentioned, with many individuals noting not just physical improvements but also enhanced emotional well-being and mental clarity.

I encourage you to document and share your own experiences with somatic exercises. Not only does this create a sense of accountability, but it also contributes to a community of support. Sharing your story can inspire others who might be facing similar challenges, offering them hope and motivation. Additionally, your feedback can help improve future resources, making these practices more accessible and effective for everyone. By creating a network of shared experiences, we can foster a supportive environment where everyone feels encouraged and empowered to pursue their well-being.

BUILDING A SUPPORTIVE COMMUNITY

When I first started practicing somatic exercises, I often felt isolated. It seemed like I was alone in my struggles with stress and pain. Then, I discovered the power of a supportive community. Having a network of people who share similar experiences and goals can make a world of difference. Shared experiences and advice are invaluable. When you connect with others who understand what you're going through, you gain insights and tips that you might have yet to consider. This exchange of advice can accelerate your progress and keep you motivated. Emotional and motivational support is another significant benefit. On days when you feel like giving up, a supportive community can lift your spirits and remind you why you started in the first place. Opportunities for learning and growth are also abundant. Engaging with others exposes you to new techniques and approaches, broadening your understanding and enhancing your practice.

Connecting with a community may seem daunting initially, but there are several ways to find and join somatic exercise groups. Online forums and social media groups are excellent starting points. Platforms like Facebook and Reddit have dedicated groups where members share their experiences, ask questions, and provide support. Local classes and workshops offer in-person interaction, allowing you to meet others face-to-face and build connections. Many community centers and wellness studios offer classes specifically focused on somatic exercises. Virtual meetups and webinars are also great options, especially if you prefer the convenience of participating from home. These online events often feature expert speakers and interactive sessions, providing a rich learning experience.

Engaging with a community offers several features that enhance your practice. Peer support and encouragement are fundamental. When you're part of a group, you receive constant feedback and motivation from others who are on a similar path. This sense of camaraderie can make your practice more enjoyable and fulfilling. Access to additional resources and events is another perk. Many communities organize special events like workshops, seminars, and retreats, providing you with opportunities to deepen your practice and learn from experts. Collaboration and sharing are also integral to a supportive community. Whether it's sharing progress updates, celebrating milestones, or collaborating on new techniques, engaging with others fosters a sense of belonging and mutual growth.

Consider sharing your personal progress and challenges to actively participate and get the most out of your community. Being open about your experiences helps you reflect on your journey and encourages others to share their insights and support. Participating in discussions and activities is another way to stay engaged. Join conversations, attend events, and contribute to group projects. Active involvement will make you feel more connected and invested in the community. Offering support and advice to others is equally important. When you help someone else, you reinforce your own understanding and create a positive, reciprocal environment. Simple acts like responding to a question or offering words of encouragement can make a big difference.

When I first joined a somatic exercise group, I hesitated to share my struggles. But as I opened up, I found that others were eager to offer advice and support. It wasn't long before I started seeing progress, both in my practice and in my emotional well-being. The sense of community kept me motivated and accountable. I realized that my journey wasn't just about personal growth; it was about contributing to a collective effort where everyone benefits. This mutual support and shared learning created a rich, nurturing environment that could not be replicated in isolation.

Joining a community might seem intimidating, but the benefits far outweigh the initial discomfort. Having a network of like-minded individuals provides a safety net of support, advice, and encouragement. Whether you're struggling with maintaining consistency, need help with specific exercises, or simply want to share your progress, a supportive community can be a game-changer. By actively participating, you not only enhance your own practice but also contribute to the growth and well-being of others. This interconnectedness fosters a sense of purpose and belonging, making your somatic journey more meaningful and rewarding.

TROUBLESHOOTING COMMON ISSUES

During my initial foray into somatic exercises, I encountered several stumbling blocks that almost derailed my progress. It's crucial to acknowledge these challenges because they are common and entirely normal. One of the most persistent issues is maintaining consistency. Life gets busy, and it can be tough to stick to a routine. Without a set schedule, it's easy to let days slip by without practice. Discomfort or pain during exercises is another frequent problem. You might experience muscle soreness or even sharp pain, which can be discouraging. Additionally, feeling unmotivated or discouraged is a hurdle many face, especially when progress seems slow or stagnates.

To maintain consistency, start by setting realistic goals and schedules. Begin with small, manageable commitments, like a 10-minute session each day. Over time, you can gradually increase the duration or complexity of your routines. Using reminders and alarms can also be incredibly helpful. Set daily reminders on your phone or calendar to prompt you to practice. This consistent nudge helps cement the habit. Finding a practice buddy for accountability can make a world of difference. When you have someone to share your progress with, it adds a layer of commitment. You can motivate each other, share tips, and celebrate milestones together.

Experiencing discomfort or pain during somatic exercises is not uncommon, but it needs to be addressed carefully to prevent injury. Proper technique is paramount. Always pay close attention to how you perform each movement. If you're unsure about your form, consider seeking guidance from instructional videos or a professional. Modifying exercises to suit your body's needs is also crucial. If a movement feels too intense, adjust it to a more comfortable range. Never push through sharp pain; it's your body's way of signaling that something is wrong. For persistent issues, consulting professionals like chiropractors, physical therapists or somatic practitioners can provide personalized advice and modifications tailored to your needs.

Staying motivated and overcoming discouragement requires a multi-faceted approach. Celebrating small milestones is a great way to keep your spirits high. Acknowledge and reward yourself for each achievement, whether it's completing a week of consistent practice or mastering a new exercise. Reflecting on personal progress can also reignite your motivation. Keep a journal where you document your experiences, noting how you feel before and after each session. This practice not only tracks your progress but also provides a tangible reminder of the benefits you're gaining. Seeking inspiration from success stories can be incredibly uplifting. Reading about others who have faced similar challenges and triumphed can renew your determination and provide practical tips for your own practice.

One of my own struggles was staying consistent with my routine amid a hectic schedule. I found that setting aside a specific time each day, just like I would for any other important appointment, made a significant difference. Treating my practice as a non-negotiable part of my day helped me stick to it. On days when I felt particularly unmotivated, I would revisit my journal to remind myself of the progress I had made and the benefits I had experienced. This simple act often provided the boost I needed to get back on track.

Addressing discomfort required me to be honest with myself about my limits. Initially, I pushed through the pain, thinking it was a sign of progress. However, I soon realized this approach was counterproductive. I started paying closer attention to my body's signals and adjusted my exercises accordingly. For instance, if a particular movement caused sharp pain, I would modify it or switch to a gentler alternative.

Motivation ebbs and flows, and that's okay. What matters is finding ways to rekindle it when it wanes. Celebrating small victories became a cornerstone of my practice. After a week of consistent practice, I would treat myself to a relaxing activity. These small rewards created positive associations with my routine, making it something I looked forward to rather than a chore. Additionally, connecting with others who shared similar goals provided a sense of camaraderie and mutual encouragement. We would share our struggles and successes, offering support and inspiration to one another.

In summary, troubleshooting common issues in somatic practice involves recognizing and addressing challenges head-on. Maintaining consistency, managing discomfort, and staying motivated are all achievable with the right strategies and mindset. By setting realistic goals, paying attention to your body's signals, and celebrating your progress, you can overcome these hurdles and continue to benefit from your practice.

CONTINUING YOUR SOMATIC PRACTICE: NEXT STEPS

One of the most important lessons I've learned in my somatic practice is the value of consistency. The long-term benefits of maintaining a regular routine are numerous and profound. Consistent practice not only helps solidify the mind-body connection but also offers ongoing relief from stress, pain, and emotional turmoil. Over time, you develop a deeper understanding of your body, gaining insights that can transform your overall well-being. Personal growth and transformation are natural outcomes of this continual engagement. Each session builds on the last, leading to incremental improvements that accumulate into significant change.

Setting new goals is a crucial aspect of maintaining an engaging and rewarding practice. As you progress, it's important to personalize your objectives based on your achievements and areas of interest. For instance, if you've successfully managed your chronic pain, you might shift your focus to enhancing emotional resilience or improving flexibility. Exploring new areas of interest keeps your practice fresh and exciting. Perhaps you'll discover a passion for somatic dance or find that integrating breathwork with movement offers new levels of relaxation. Setting both short-term and long-term goals ensures that you have immediate milestones to celebrate and larger objectives to strive towards. These goals provide direction and motivation, encouraging you to push your boundaries and explore the full potential of somatic exercises.

Sustaining a lifelong practice requires integrating somatic exercises into your daily life. Finding ways to incorporate these practices into your routine makes them a natural part of your day rather than an additional task. Simple activities like mindful walking or taking a few minutes for breathwork during breaks can make a significant difference. Staying curious and open to new techniques is also vital. The field of somatic exercises is continually evolving, with new methods and insights emerging regularly. Being open to experimenting with different approaches keeps your practice dynamic and effective. Building a supportive network for ongoing encouragement can provide the motivation and accountability needed to maintain your practice. Whether it's joining a local group, participating in online forums, or having a practice buddy, a supportive network can make the journey more enjoyable and sustainable.

As you continue your somatic practice, remember that the journey is ongoing. There will always be new goals to set, new techniques to explore, and new levels of understanding to achieve. Embrace this continual growth and let it guide you towards greater well-being and personal transformation.

8

QUICK AND EFFECTIVE 10-MINUTE ROUTINES

One morning, I struggled to shake off the grogginess that clung to me like a heavy blanket. Despite my best efforts, my energy levels were low, and my mood was flat. Determined to turn my day around, I decided to try a 10-minute morning routine I had read about. As I moved through the gentle stretches and light cardio, I felt my body waking up and my mind clearing. By the end of the routine, I was energized and ready to face the day with a positive mindset. This experience highlighted the power of a morning routine and how it can set a positive tone for the rest of the day.

10-MINUTE MORNING ROUTINE FOR ENERGY

Starting your day with somatic exercises can be transformative. This 10-minute routine will invigorate both your body and mind, boosting your energy and mood to set you up for a productive and positive day.

1. Standing Forward Bend with Overhead Stretch

- **Instructions**:
    - Stand tall with your feet hip-width apart.
    - Inhale as you reach your arms overhead, stretching your entire body.
    - Exhale as you fold forward, reaching for your toes in a standing forward bend.
    - Hold the position for a few deep breaths, feeling the stretch in your hamstrings and lower back.
- **Cue**: Focus on slow, controlled movements and deep breathing to fully awaken your muscles.

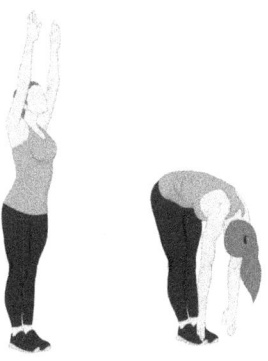

2. Cat-Cow Stretch

- **Instructions**:
    - Get down on your hands and knees, with your wrists aligned under your shoulders and knees under your hips.
    - Inhale as you round your spine, tucking your chin to your chest (Cat pose).

QUICK AND EFFECTIVE 10-MINUTE ROUTINES | 143

- Exhale as you arch your back, lifting your head and tailbone toward the ceiling (Cow pose).
- Continue this movement for one minute, coordinating your breath with each motion.
- **Cue**: Move fluidly through the stretch, feeling each motion wake up your spine and muscles.

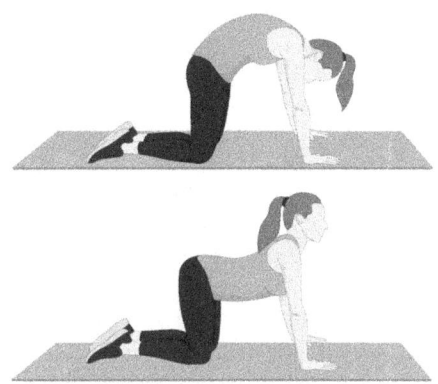

3. Standing Spinal Twists

- **Instructions**:
    - Stand with your feet hip-width apart.
    - Gently twist your torso to the right, allowing your arms to swing naturally.
    - Then twist to the left.
    - Alternate sides for one minute to release tension in your back and shoulders.
- **Cue**: Keep your movements loose and natural, allowing your arms to swing freely with each twist.

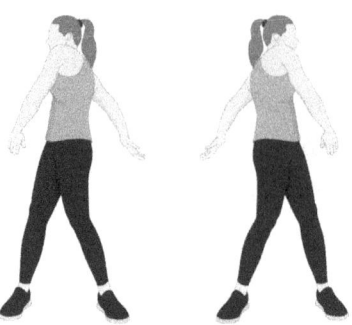

4. Light Cardio: Marching in Place and Gentle Jogging

- **Instructions**:
    - Start by marching in place for one minute, gradually lifting your knees higher with each step.
    - Swing your arms actively to engage your upper body.
    - After a minute, transition into gentle jogging in place, or continue marching if jogging is uncomfortable.
    - Continue for another minute to increase circulation and boost your energy levels.
- **Cue**: Focus on keeping your body light and active, breathing deeply as you move.

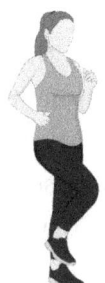 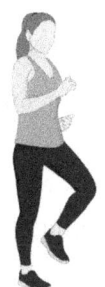

5. Forward Fold and Roll Up

- **Instructions**:
    - Return to the standing forward bend, allowing your body to hang loosely.
    - Slowly roll up to standing, one vertebra at a time.
    - Once standing, take a few deep breaths with your arms overhead, feeling the energy flow through your body.
- **Cue**: Use this final stretch to release any remaining tension and ground yourself for the day ahead.

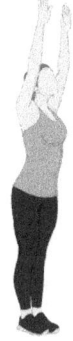 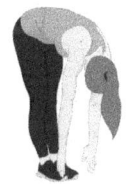

Tips for Consistency

- **Set a Regular Wake-Up Time**: Choose a time that allows you to fit in your 10-minute routine without feeling rushed.
- **Prepare Your Space**: Lay out your exercise mat, props, and comfortable clothing the night before to make it easier to start your routine in the morning.
- **Use Alarms and Reminders**: Set an alarm or reminder on your phone to wake up and start your routine. Consistency is key to making this a habit.

Quick Tip:

Incorporating this 10-minute routine daily can boost your energy, improve focus, and elevate your mood. The more consistently you practice, the more benefits you'll experience throughout your day.

10-MINUTE LUNCHTIME STRESS-BUSTER ROUTINE

Taking a break during your day for somatic exercises can be a game-changer. Midday exercises offer a chance to reset and recharge, reducing stress and increasing productivity. This simple 10-minute routine can release tension, lower stress hormones, and improve your focus for the rest of the day.

1. Shoulder Rolls

- **Instructions:** Sit comfortably in your chair with your feet flat on the floor. Roll your shoulders forward in a circular motion for about 30 seconds, then reverse the direction and roll them backward.
- **Cue:** Keep the movements slow and smooth, focusing on releasing tension in your upper back and shoulders.

QUICK AND EFFECTIVE 10-MINUTE ROUTINES | 147

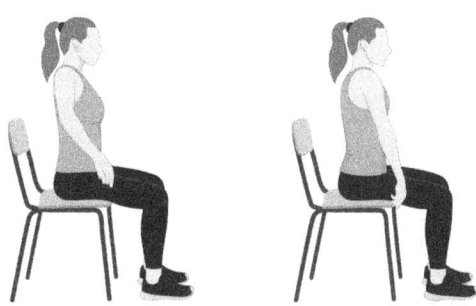

2. Seated Spinal Twists

- **Instructions:** Sit up straight, place your right hand on the back of your chair, and your left hand on your right knee. Gently twist your torso to the right, looking over your shoulder. Hold for a few deep breaths. Repeat on the other side.
- **Cue:** Focus on feeling the stretch along your spine and the release of tension as you breathe deeply.

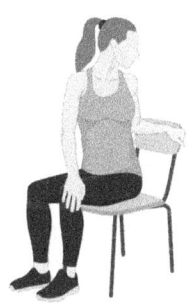

3. Box Breathing

- **Instructions:** Sit with your back straight and close your eyes. Inhale deeply for 4 seconds, hold your breath for 4 seconds, exhale for 4 seconds, and hold again for 4 seconds. Repeat for 1-2 minutes.
- **Cue:** Focus on your breath and how it feels to calm your body and mind.

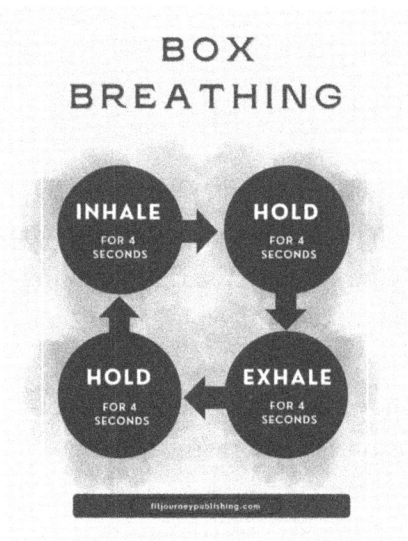

4. Shoulder Shrugs

- **Instructions:** Lift your shoulders up towards your ears, hold for a few seconds, then release them down with an exhale. Repeat this movement 5-10 times.
- **Cue:** Focus on releasing any built-up tension in your shoulders with each exhale.

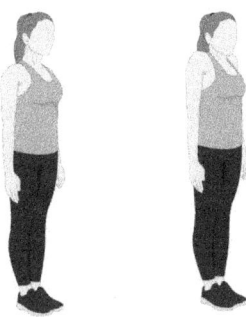

5. Seated Cat-Cow Stretch

- **Instructions:** Sit on the edge of your chair with your hands on your knees. Inhale as you arch your back, lifting your chest and looking up (Cow pose). Exhale as you round your spine, tucking your chin to your chest (Cat pose). Continue for 1 minute, coordinating your breath with each motion.
- **Cue:** Move fluidly between the two poses, using your breath to enhance the stretch and relieve tension in your spine.

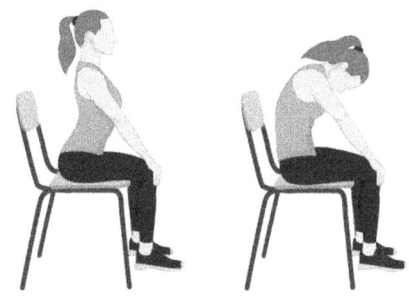

6. Seated Forward Fold Stretch

- **Instructions:** While seated, widen your legs slightly, hinge at your hips, and fold forward. Allow your hands to reach toward the floor, and let your head hang heavy. Take a few deep breaths in this position.
- **Cue:** Relax your neck and lower back, feeling the stretch in your hamstrings and the release of tension.

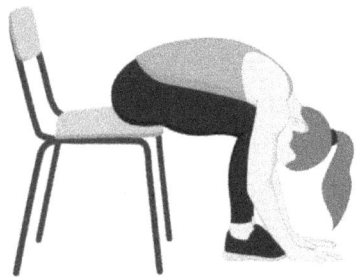

Mindfulness Techniques

After completing the physical exercises, take a moment to incorporate mindfulness into your routine.

- **Body Scan:** Close your eyes and take a few deep breaths. Bring your awareness to your body, starting at your feet and moving upward. Notice any areas of tension and consciously release them.
- **Focused Breathing:** Throughout the exercises, focus on the sensation of the air entering and leaving your body. This not only calms your mind but also enhances the physical benefits by promoting better oxygen flow and relaxation.

Quick Tip:

Consistent practice of these exercises throughout the week will help reduce stress, improve focus, and increase resilience to daily pressures. Incorporate this routine whenever you feel overwhelmed or need a mental and physical reset.

10-MINUTE EVENING ROUTINE FOR RELAXATION AND SLEEP

As the day winds down, our bodies and minds crave a sense of calm to transition into restful sleep. An evening routine centered around somatic exercises can be a powerful tool for unwinding and preparing for the night ahead. The benefits of evening relaxation are profound. By engaging in mindful movements and gentle stretches, you can release the tension accumulated throughout the day, helping to lower cortisol levels and promote a sense of tranquility. This process not only eases you into sleep but also improves its quality, making it deeper and more restorative.

This 10-minute evening routine, centered around gentle somatic exercises, can help release the day's tension and prepare you for a deeper, more restorative sleep.

1. Legs Up the Wall Pose

- **Instructions**:
    - Find a clear wall space. Sit sideways with one hip touching the wall, then swing your legs up as you lie back, allowing your legs to rest against the wall.
    - Hold this position for a few minutes, breathing deeply and allowing your body to settle.
- **Cue**: Focus on feeling the tension release from your legs and back as you breathe deeply.

- **Benefits**: This pose helps reduce swelling in the legs, calms the nervous system, and promotes relaxation.

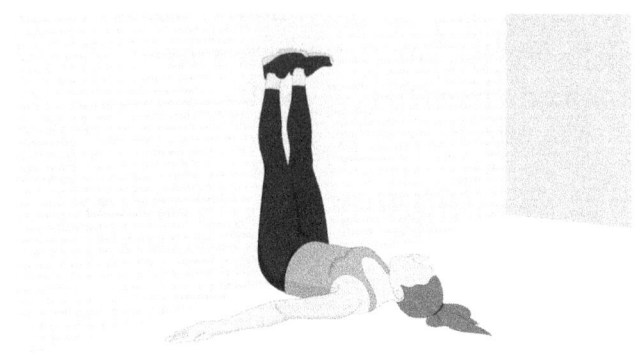

2. Reclining Bound Ankle Pose

- **Instructions**:
    - Lie on your back with your knees bent and the soles of your feet touching, allowing your knees to fall open to the sides.
    - You can place pillows or blocks under your knees for added support.
    - Hold this position for a few minutes, focusing on deep diaphragmatic breathing.
- **Cue**: Breathe deeply into your belly, allowing your hips and groin to gently release tension.
- **Benefits**: Opens the hips and groin, releases tension, and encourages deep relaxation through focused breathing.

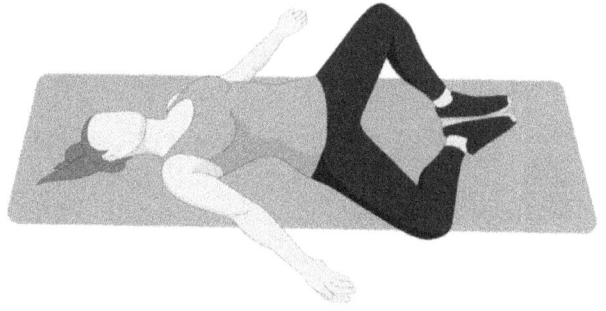

3. Gentle Spinal Twists

- **Instructions**:
    - Lie on your back with your knees bent and feet flat on the floor.
    - Drop your knees to one side while keeping your shoulders grounded, and turn your head in the opposite direction.
    - Hold this position for a few deep breaths, then switch sides.
- **Cue**: Allow your breath to guide the movement and feel the stretch along your spine and hips.
- **Benefits**: Releases tension in the back and hips, improves spinal flexibility, and promotes digestion.

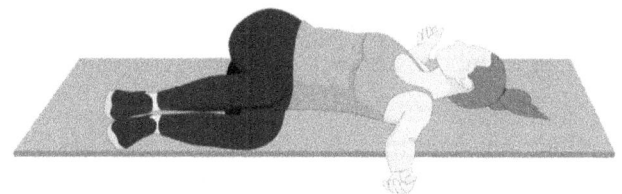

Relaxation Techniques

After completing the stretches, take a moment to practice deep breathing.

- **Deep Breathing Exercise**:
    - Sit or lie down comfortably, close your eyes, and take a deep breath in through your nose, allowing your abdomen to expand.
    - Hold your breath for a moment, then exhale slowly through your mouth, feeling your body relax with each exhale.
    - Repeat this process for a few minutes, focusing on the sensation of your breath and letting go of any remaining tension.
- **Cue**: Visualize releasing stress with each exhale as your body and mind relax.

Sleep Hygiene Tips

To optimize your evening routine and enhance your sleep quality, consider these helpful tips:

- **Create a Calming Environment**:
    - Dim the lights in your room an hour before bed to signal your body that it's time to wind down. Soft, warm lighting can create a soothing atmosphere.
- **Avoid Screens Before Bed**:
    - The blue light emitted from phones, tablets, and computers can interfere with your body's natural sleep-wake cycle. Try to put away electronic devices at least an hour before bedtime.

- **Engage in Relaxing Activities**:
    - Instead of screen time, engage in calming activities such as reading, taking a warm bath, or practicing your somatic evening routine.
- **Establish a Consistent Sleep Schedule**:
    - Going to bed and waking up at the same time every day helps regulate your internal clock, making it easier to fall asleep and wake up naturally.

Quick Tip:

Develop a pre-sleep ritual that includes this evening somatic routine. Over time, this will signal your body that it's time to rest, making the transition to sleep smoother and more effective.

5-MINUTE QUICK OFFICE BREAK EXERCISES

During a hectic workday, taking short exercise breaks can be incredibly beneficial. Sitting for long periods can cause physical tension, especially in the neck, shoulders, and lower back. This tension not only brings discomfort but also affects your ability to focus and be productive. Short, regular breaks for movement can help reduce this physical strain and enhance your mental clarity. When you step away from your desk and move your body, you give your mind a chance to reset. This can lead to improved concentration and better decision-making when you return to your tasks.

A quick 5-minute routine can do wonders to alleviate tension and refresh your mind. You don't need much space or any special equipment—just a few minutes of your time. Incorporate standing movements to get your blood flowing and increase your energy levels.

1. **Standing Forward Bend with Overhead Stretch**

    - **Instructions**:
        - Stand tall with your feet hip-width apart.
        - Inhale as you reach your arms overhead, stretching your entire body.
        - Exhale as you fold forward, reaching for your toes in a standing forward bend.
        - Hold this position for a few deep breaths, feeling the stretch in your hamstrings and lower back.
    - **Cue**: Focus on slow, controlled movements and deep breathing to stretch and relax your muscles.

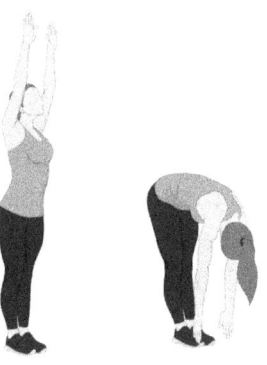

2. **Standing Calf Raises**

    - **Instructions**:
        - Stand with your feet a comfortable distance apart.
        - Rise onto the balls of your feet, lifting your heels off the ground.
        - Hold for a moment, then lower your heels back down.
        - Repeat this movement several times.

- **Cue**: Engage your core for balance and focus on improving circulation in your legs.
- **Benefits**: Calf raises help improve circulation and reduce the stiffness that comes from sitting for long periods.

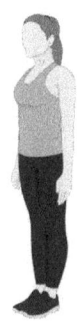 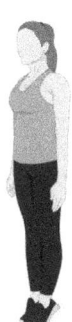

3. Chair Twists

- **Instructions**:
    - Sit with your feet firmly planted on the ground and your back straight.
    - Place your left hand on the back of the chair and your right hand on your left knee.
    - Gently twist your torso to the left, looking over your shoulder.
    - Hold for a few breaths, then return to the center and repeat on the other side.
- **Cue**: Keep your spine straight and twist gently, focusing on releasing tension in your back and spine.
- **Benefits**: Chair twists help relieve tension in the spine, increase flexibility, and improve mobility.

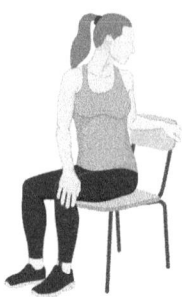

Incorporate Breaks into Your Workday

- **Set Regular Timers**:
    - Use your phone or a desktop app to set reminders to take a movement break every hour. Even a few minutes of stretching or movement can improve focus and reduce stress.
- **Take a Moment to Reset**:
    - During each break, step away from your desk, do some stretches, and take a few deep breaths. This helps clear your mind and prepares you to return to work with renewed focus and energy.
- **Encourage Movement in the Workplace**:
    - Share these exercises with your colleagues and encourage them to take breaks, too. Consider suggesting a designated area for stretching and movement in the office to promote health and wellness at work.

Quick Tip:

Incorporating short, regular movement breaks into your day can reduce physical discomfort, boost your energy, and improve your focus. A few minutes of movement can make a significant difference in how you feel and perform throughout the day.

10-MINUTE TRAVEL-FRIENDLY SOMATIC EXERCISES

Traveling can make it challenging to maintain a consistent exercise routine. The disruptions to your schedule, limited space, and unfamiliar environments all contribute to the difficulty. I remember one trip where I found myself in a tiny hotel room with barely enough space to stretch my arms, let alone exercise. The stress of traveling left me feeling disoriented and drained. Yet, I discovered that with a bit of creativity and determination, it was possible to stay active and energized, even on the go.

1. Seated Leg Lifts

- **Instructions**:
    - Sit on the edge of a chair with your back straight and feet flat on the floor.
    - Lift one leg straight in front of you and hold for a few seconds, then lower it back down.
    - Repeat on the other leg. Continue alternating legs for 1-2 minutes.

- **Cue**: Engage your core and keep your movements controlled. This exercise targets your lower abs and quadriceps.
- **Benefits**: Helps maintain muscle tone and flexibility even when confined to a small space.

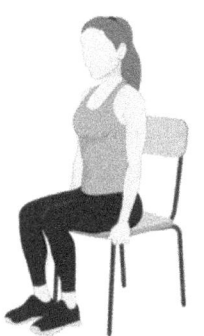 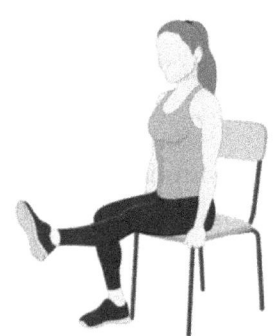

2. Standing Side Stretches

- **Instructions**:
    - Stand up with your feet hip-width apart.
    - Raise your arms overhead, clasp your hands together, and gently lean to one side.
    - Hold the stretch for a few breaths, then switch to the other side.
- **Cue**: Keep your core engaged and avoid overextending. Focus on feeling the stretch along your side body.
- **Benefits**: Opens up the torso and alleviates tension in the back and shoulders, especially helpful after long hours of sitting.

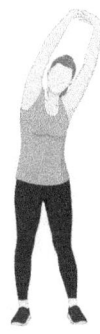

3. Ankle Circles

- **Instructions**:
    - Sit or stand with your feet flat on the floor.
    - Lift one foot off the ground and rotate your ankle in a circular motion, first clockwise, then counterclockwise.
    - Repeat with the other ankle.
- **Cue**: Make slow, controlled circles, focusing on improving circulation and flexibility in your ankles.
- **Benefits**: Improves circulation in the lower legs, reducing stiffness and swelling commonly experienced during travel.

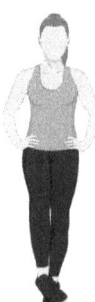 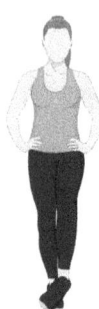

Additional Tips for Staying Active While Traveling

- **Use Hotel Gyms**:
    - If your hotel has a gym, take advantage of it. A short session on the treadmill or using available equipment can make a big difference in maintaining your fitness routine.
- **Incorporate Walking**:
    - Opt for walking whenever possible. Walking tours are a great way to explore a new city while staying active. You can also explore nearby parks or nature trails to combine exercise with sightseeing.
- **Set a Daily Routine**:
    - Choose a specific time each day for your exercise routine—whether it's in the morning before your day gets busy or in the evening to unwind. Set a reminder on your phone to stay on track.
- **Plan Ahead**:
    - Before your trip, write down a few simple routines that you can do in different settings (hotel room, park, airport lounge). Having a plan will help you stay consistent, no matter where you are.

Quick Tip:

Consistency is key. Even on a busy travel schedule, taking just 10 minutes a day to move your body can make a huge difference in how you feel and perform. Use this travel-friendly routine to stay energized and ready for your next adventure.

10-MINUTE WEEKEND WIND-DOWN ROUTINE

Weekends should be a time to relax and recharge, but often they become filled with errands and obligations. Taking time to unwind with somatic exercises can help you truly disconnect from the week's stress and prepare your body and mind for the upcoming week. When you give yourself permission to relax, you reduce stress and rejuvenate your energy levels. This not only improves your mood but also enhances your ability to tackle the demands of the new week with a fresh perspective.

Incorporating gentle yoga-inspired stretches and deep breathing exercises will ease you into a calm state, helping you recharge for the week ahead.

1. Child's Pose

- **Instructions**:
    - Begin by kneeling on the floor with your big toes touching and your knees spread apart.
    - Sit back on your heels, stretch your arms forward, and lower your torso between your thighs.
    - Rest your forehead on the mat and hold this position for a few deep breaths.
- **Cue**: Allow your hips and shoulders to relax as you breathe deeply, feeling the gentle stretch in your hips, thighs, and ankles.

- **Benefits**: Stretches the hips, thighs, and ankles while calming the mind and relieving stress.

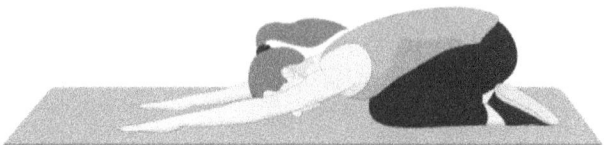

2. Supine Twists

- **Instructions**:
    - Lie on your back with your knees bent and feet flat on the floor.
    - Extend your arms out to the sides in a T position.
    - Drop your knees to one side while keeping your shoulders grounded.
    - Hold the position for a few breaths, then switch sides.
- **Cue**: Focus on keeping your shoulders on the ground as you twist, releasing tension in your spine and lower back.
- **Benefits**: Helps to release tension in the lower back and hips while improving spinal flexibility.

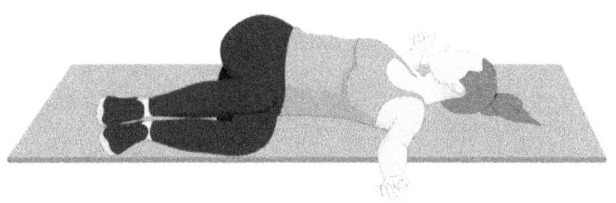

3. Happy Baby Pose

- **Instructions**:
    - Lie on your back and draw your knees towards your chest.

- Grab the outer edges of your feet with your hands, keeping your ankles stacked over your knees.
- Gently rock side to side, massaging your lower back against the floor.
- **Cue**: Relax into the movement, focusing on the stretch in your hips and inner thighs while gently rocking.
- **Benefits**: Stretches the inner thighs, hips, and groin while promoting a playful, joyful sense of lightness.

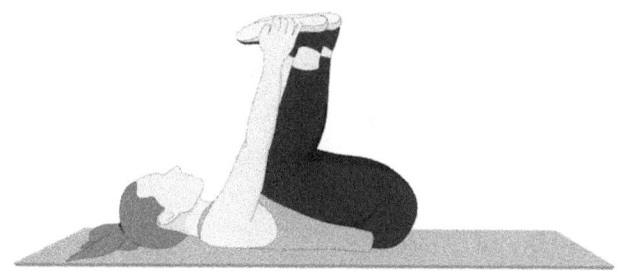

Incorporate Deep Breathing

- **Instructions**: While lying in Happy Baby Pose, begin practicing deep breathing to enhance relaxation.
    - **Deep Breathing**: Inhale deeply through your nose, letting your belly rise.
    - Hold for a moment, then exhale slowly through your mouth, feeling your belly fall.
    - Continue this deep, mindful breathing for several minutes.
- **Cue**: Focus on the rhythm of your breath, allowing each inhale and exhale to bring deeper relaxation.
- **Benefits**: Calms the mind, reduces stress, and helps release any lingering tension.

Create a Relaxing Environment

- **Music**: Play calming music or nature sounds, such as gentle waves or soft piano melodies, to create a peaceful atmosphere.
- **Aromatherapy**: Use essential oils like lavender, chamomile, or sandalwood to enhance relaxation. You can diffuse the oils or apply them to your wrists or temples.
- **Nature**: If possible, practice outside in a serene setting like a garden or park. Being in nature can amplify the calming effects of your routine, offering fresh air and natural surroundings to soothe your mind.

Tips for Consistency

- **Set a Regular Time**: Incorporate this routine into your weekend to create a sanctuary of relaxation. Try practicing at the same time each weekend to make it a consistent, cherished part of your routine.
- **Mind-Body Connection**: Focus on the present moment during your practice, letting go of distractions and allowing yourself to fully relax.

Quick Tip:

Taking time for yourself with this wind-down routine helps reset your mind and body, making you more resilient to stress and better equipped for the week ahead.

KEEPING THE JOURNEY ALIVE

Now that you have all the tools you need to **ease stress and anxiety, manage chronic pain, and build emotional resilience**, it's time to share what you've learned and help others find the same relief.

By simply leaving your honest review on Amazon, you'll guide other **Health and Wellness Advocates** to the information they need, and help them discover the power of **Somatic Exercises**. Your review can make a difference for someone just starting their journey, just as you did.

Thank you for your support. **Our mind-body connection** thrives when we pass on our knowledge—and you're helping me spread that message to more people each day.

Scan the QR code to leave your review on Amazon

CONCLUSION

As we conclude this guide, I want to emphasize the transformative potential of somatic exercises. These practices are not just accessible, enjoyable, and effective, but they also hold the power to significantly improve your life. Whether you're a beginner or not, amidst the hustle and bustle of life, you can find relief from stress and anxiety, manage pain, and build emotional resilience. With just 10 minutes a day, you can set in motion profound changes in your well-being.

Throughout this book, we've explored the foundations of somatic exercises. We've learned how they focus on internal body awareness and the mind-body connection. We discussed how these exercises differ from traditional workouts, emphasizing sensory awareness and neuromuscular control. We delved into the science behind somatic exercises, understanding how they tap into neuroplasticity to form new, healthier movement patterns.

We've covered somatic routines for various needs—stress and anxiety relief, pain management, and boosting emotional resilience. Each chapter provided step-by-step instructions, practical examples, and scientific backing to ensure you have a comprehensive understanding of the exercises and their benefits.

One of the key takeaways I hope you remember is the incredible power of mindful movement. By paying attention to your body, you can alleviate physical tension and improve your mental clarity. Another important point is the role of breathwork. Simple breathing techniques can instantly calm your mind and reduce stress. Remember the importance of consistency. Even short, daily practices can lead to lasting results.

In my journey, I've spent over 20 years teaching health and physical education, guiding students toward healthier lives. I wrote this book because I wanted to extend that guidance to you. I remember beginning my journey with somatic exercises after a stressful day. The relief I felt was profound and immediate, and it opened my eyes to the potential of these practices. This personal experience, combined with my professional background, motivated me to create an easy-to-follow and impactful guide.

As you move forward, I encourage you to integrate these exercises into your daily routine. Start small. Commit to a few minutes each day. Track your progress and celebrate your achievements. Use the techniques we've discussed—body scans, mindful breathing, gentle stretches—to navigate stressful moments and manage pain.

I also want to express my heartfelt gratitude. Thank you for allowing me to be a part of your journey towards better health. Your willingness to explore somatic exercises is the first step towards a more balanced and fulfilling life. Remember, you have the tools and support needed to master these practices. Trust the process and be patient with yourself. You are not alone in this journey, and your efforts are deeply appreciated.

In conclusion, I believe in the power of somatic exercises to change lives. I've seen it in my own life and in the lives of my students. Now, it's your turn. Embrace these practices, and let them guide you towards a healthier, happier, and more balanced life.

Thank you for joining me on this journey.

REFERENCES

A Brief Overview & History of Somatics. (n.d.). Somatic Education. https://somatics.org/about/introduction/overview-history

Anytime Fitness. (n.d.). What are somatic exercises? A guide for beginners. https://www.anytimefitness.com/ccc/care/what-are-somatic-exercises-a-guide-for-beginners/

ASI Recreation. (2021). The importance of tracking your fitness progress. https://asirecreation.org/recreport/special-feature/592-the-importance-of-tracking-your-fitness-progress

Brain First Institute. (n.d.). Somatic awareness: The science of connecting mind and body. https://www.brainfirstinstitute.com/blog/somatic-awareness-the-science-of-connecting-mind-and-body

By Repose. (n.d.). Somatic therapy techniques to combat insomnia: A holistic approach. https://byrepose.com/journal/somatic-therapy-techniques-to-combat-insomnia/

Charlie Health. (2023). Try these somatic exercises to improve your mental health. https://www.charliehealth.com/post/somatic-exercises-for-mental-health

ChallengeRunner. (n.d.). Free online fitness challenge platform. https://www.challengerunner.com/

Effects of physical exercise on neuroplasticity and brain function. (2020). National Center for Biotechnology Information. https://www.ncbi.nlm.nih.gov/pmc/articles/PMC7752270/

Effectiveness of diaphragmatic breathing for reducing stress. (2019). PubMed. https://pubmed.ncbi.nlm.nih.gov/31436595/

Frontiers in Nutrition. (2021). The impact of nutrients on mental health and well-being. https://www.frontiersin.org/journals/nutrition/articles/10.3389/fnut.2021.656290/full

Healthline. (n.d.). A daily 5-minute stretching routine that everyone needs. https://www.healthline.com/health/fitness-exercise/daily-stretching-routine

Healthline. (n.d.). 13 benefits of working out in the morning. https://www.healthline.com/health/exercise-fitness/working-out-in-the-morning

HeartMath. (n.d.). Heart-focused breathing. https://www.heartmath.org/articles-of-the-heart/the-math-of-heartmath/heart-focused-breathing/

International Somatic Movement Education & Therapy Association. (n.d.). ISMETA: Home. https://ismeta.org/

Kirstein, M. (2023). 7 best somatic breathwork exercises for stress-relief. https://www.monakirstein.com/somatic-breathwork/

Live Science. (2023). Do 30-day fitness challenges actually work? https://www.livescience.com/do-30-day-fitness-challenges-work

Mindful. (2023). How to manage stress with mindfulness and meditation. https://www.mindful.org/how-to-manage-stress-with-mindfulness-and-meditation/

Mindfulness-based stress reduction: A non-invasive treatment. (2012). National Center for Biotechnology Information. https://www.ncbi.nlm.nih.gov/pmc/articles/PMC3336928/

Moving with pain: What principles from somatic practices can teach us. (2021). National Center for Biotechnology Information. https://www.ncbi.nlm.nih.gov/pmc/articles/PMC7868595/

Nerd Fitness. (n.d.). Stay in shape while traveling (5 workouts). https://www.nerdfitness.com/blog/how-to-stay-in-shape-while-traveling/

Nivati. (2022). 12 best workplace stress relief techniques for the office. https://www.nivati.com/blog/12-best-workplace-stress-relief-tips-techniques

Positive Psychology. (2023). 13 self-reflection worksheets & templates to use in therapy. https://positivepsychology.com/reflection-journal-worksheets/

Positive Psychology. (2023). Guided imagery in therapy: 20 powerful scripts and examples. https://positivepsychology.com/guided-imagery-scripts/

Prime Mind. (2023). 14 benefits of guided meditation backed by science. https://primedmind.com/benefits-of-guided-meditation/

Somatic experiencing – Effectiveness and key factors of a somatic-based therapy. (2021). National Center for Biotechnology Information. https://www.ncbi.nlm.nih.gov/pmc/articles/PMC8276649/

Somatic movement center. (n.d.). Clinical somatics testimonials. https://somaticmovementcenter.com/somatics-testimonials/

Somatic movement center. (n.d.). How to get rid of your chronic neck pain: Pandiculate! https://somaticmovementcenter.com/neck-pain/

Somatic movement center. (n.d.). Somatics exercise for back pain - Learn at home. https://somaticmovementcenter.com/somatics-exercise-for-back-pain/

Somatic movement center. (n.d.). Sensations you may notice when beginning your clinical somatics practice. https://somaticmovementcenter.com/sensations/

The effects of acute exercise on mood, cognition, neuroplasticity. (2018). National Center for Biotechnology Information. https://www.ncbi.nlm.nih.gov/pmc/articles/PMC5928534/

The YMCA of Pierce and Kitsap Counties. (2023). Unveiling 10 science-backed secrets to staying motivated at the gym. https://www.ymcapkc.org/blog/unveiling-10-science-backed-secrets-staying-motivated-gym

Somatic therapy and the mind-body connection. (2023). Psychology Today. https://www.psychologytoday.com/us/blog/click-here-for-happiness/202309/somatic-therapy-and-the-mind-body-connection

www.ingramcontent.com/pod-product-compliance
Lightning Source LLC
Chambersburg PA
CBHW062124040426
42337CB00044B/3946